Handbook of Critical Care

Third Edition

Handbook of Critical Care

Third Edition

Editor
Jesse B. Hall
University of Chicago
Chicago, IL
USA

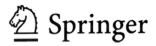 Springer

Editor
Jesse B. Hall
Department of Medicine MC 6076
Section of Pulmonary and Critical Care Medicine
University of Chicago
5841, South Maryland Avenue
Chicago, IL 60637
USA
jhall@medicine.uchicago.edu

ISBN 978-1-84882-723-3   e-ISBN 978-1-84882-724-0
DOI 10.1007/978-1-84882-724-0
Springer Dordrecht Heidelberg London New York

Library of Congress Control Number: 2009928774

Springer is part of Springer Science+Business Media (www.springer.com)

Contents

Author biographies   vii

Abbreviations   ix

1 An approach to critical care   1

2 Analgesia and sedation in the intensive care unit   7

3 The cardiovascular system   15

4 The respiratory system   53

5 Acute renal failure   97

6 Neurologic emergencies   109

7 The endocrine system   141

8 Gastrointestinal disorders   155

9 Infection and inflammation   171

10 Hematologic emergencies   185

11 Nutritional support   197

12 Physical injury   203

13 Toxicology   237

14 Scoring systems   251

15 Obstetric emergencies   255

Index   263

Author biographies

Editor
Jesse B Hall MD is Professor of Medicine, Anesthesia and Critical Care, and Section Chief of Pulmonary and Critical Care Medicine at the University of Chicago. Dr Hall's clinical, teaching, and research interests include outcomes from critical illness, pharmacology in the intensive care unit (ICU), respiratory failure, and shock. He has worked throughout his career to develop the ICU not only as a place for exemplary care, but also as a laboratory for clinical investigation and a classroom for bedside teaching.

Contributing authors
Brian Gehlbach MD graduated from Washington University School of Medicine and underwent his residency and fellowship training at the University of Chicago, where he now serves as Assistant Professor of Medicine in the Section of Pulmonary and Critical Care. His research interests include analysis of outcomes of critical care and the study of sleep in the critically ill.

John Kress MD is a graduate of St Louis University School of Medicine. He completed a residency in Anesthesiology at the University of Chicago, followed by a residency in Internal Medicine and a fellowship in Pulmonary and Critical Care Medicine, also at the University of Chicago. He is currently Associate Professor of Medicine in the Section of Pulmonary and Critical Care Medicine at the University of Chicago. His clinical interests include attending in the medical ICU. His research interests include outcomes in critical care and sedation of mechanically ventilated patients in the ICU.

Imre Noth MD is a graduate of the University of Arizona College of Medicine. He completed an internal medicine residency at the University of California, Davis, and went on to subspecialty training at the University of Chicago in Pulmonary and Critical Care Medicine. His clinical interests include adult pulmonary medicine as well as attending in the medical ICU at the University of Chicago.

List of abbreviations

ABC	airway, breathing, circulation
ACE	angiotensin-converting enzyme
ACEI	angiotensin-converting enzyme inhibitor
ACh	acetylcholine
ACTH	adrenocorticotropic hormone
ADH	antidiuretic hormone
AF	atrial fibrillation
AFE	amniotic fluid embolism
AHRF	acute hypoxemic respiratory failure
ALI	acute lung injury
ALT	alanine aminotransferase
AMD	airway management devide
AMI	acute myocardial infarction
APACHE	Acute Physiology and Chronic Health Evaluation
APTT	activated partial thromboplastin time
ARDS	acute respiratory distress syndrome
ARDSnet	acute respiratory distress syndrome network
AST	aspartate transaminase
ATP	adenosine triphosphate
aVF	arteriovenous fistula
aVL	accessory vein ligation
AV	atrioventricular
BP	blood pressure
BSA	body surface area
BUN	blood urea nitrogen
BV	blood volume
cAMP	cyclic adenosine $3'$-$5'$-monophosphate
CBF	cerebral blood flow
CI	cardiac index
CK	creatine kinase
CMV	controlled mandatory ventilation; cytomegalovirus
CNS	central nervous system
CO	carbon monoxide; cardiac output
CO_2	carbon dioxide
COPD	chronic obstructive pulmonary disease
CPAP	continuous positive airway pressure
CPP	cerebral perfusion pressure

CPR	cardiopulmonary resuscitation
CSF	cerebrospinal fluid
CT	computed tomography
CVA	cerebrovascular accident
CVP	central venous pressure
DC	direct current
DDAVP	deamino-D-arginine vasopressin
DI	diabetes insipidus
DIC	disseminated intravascular coagulation
DKA	diabetic ketoacidosis
DO_2	tissue oxygen delivery
2,3-DPG	2,3-diphosphoglycerate
DPL	diagnostic peritoneal lavage
DVT	deep venous thrombosis
EBV	Epstein–Barr virus
ECF	extracellular fluid
ECG	electrocardiogram
ECL	enterochromaffin like
EDTA	ethylenediaminetetraacetic acid
EEG	electroencephalogram
EMG	electromyogram
ERCP	endoscopic retrograde cholangiopancreatography
ETT	endotracheal tube
FDP	fibrin degradation product
FiO_2	fraction of inspired oxygen in a gas mixture
FFP	fresh frozen plasma
FRC	functional residual capacity
GCS	Glasgow Coma Scale
GTN	glyceryl trinitrate
HAS	human albumin solution
Hb	hemoglobin
HbCO	carboxyhemoglobin
HbO_2	oxyhemoglobin
HELLP	hemolysis, elevated liver enzymes, and low platelets
HIV	human immunodeficiency virus
HR	heart rate
hTIG	human tetanus immunoglobulin
ICP	intracranial pressure
ICU	intensive care unit

IgG	immunoglobulin G
IgM	immunoglobulin M
INR	international normalized ratio
IPPV	intermittent positive pressure ventilation
IUGR	intrauterine growth retardation
IV	intravenous
LAHB	left anterior hemiblock
LBBB	left bundle-branch block
LDH	lactate dehydrogenase
LEMS	Lambert–Eaton myasthenic syndrome
LPHB	left posterior hemiblock
LV	left ventricle
LVEDV	left ventricular end-diastolic volume
LVSW	left ventricular stroke work
MAP	mean arterial pressure
MDAC	multiple-dose activated charcoal
MDR	multidrug resistant
MEP	maximum expiratory pressure
metHb	methemoglobin
MODS	multiple organ dysfunction syndrome
MPAP	mean pulmonary artery pressure
MRI	magnetic resonance imaging
MRSA	methicillin-resistant *Staphylococcus aureus*
MU	mega-unit
NSAID	nonsteroidal anti-inflammatory drug
EDM	esophageal Doppler monitoring
PAC	pulmonary artery catheter
$PaCO_2$	partial pressure of carbon dioxide
PAFC	pulmonary artery flotation catheter
PaO_2	partial pressure of oxygen
PAP	pulmonary artery pressure
PAWP	pulmonary artery wedge pressure
PCV	pressure-controlled ventilation
PE	pulmonary embolism
PEEP	positive end-expiratory pressure
PEFR	peak expiratory flow rate
PIFR	peak inspiratory flow rate
pK_a	acid dissociation constant
PPIs	proton-pump inhibitors

PT	prothrombin time
PTH	parathyroid hormone
PTT	partial thromboplastin time
PVR	peripheral vascular resistance
$\dot{Q}$	perfusion; cardiac output
$\dot{Q}s/\dot{Q}t$	shunt fraction
RBBB	right bundle-branch block
RBC	red blood cell
RCA	right coronary artery
RSV	respiratory syncytial virus
rT_3	reverse triiodothyronine
rtPA	recombinant tissue-type plasminogen activator
RV	reserve volume; right ventricle
RVEDV	right ventricular end-diastolic volume
RVSW	right ventricular stroke work
SaO_2	arterial oxygen saturation
SBP	systolic blood pressure
SCI	spinal cord injury
SIADH	syndrome of inappropriate antidiuretic hormone secretion
SIMV	synchronized intermittent mandatory ventilation
SIRS	systemic inflammatory response syndrome
SLE	systemic lupus erythematosus
SMX	sulfamethoxazole
SV	stroke volume
SVC	superior vena cava
SVR	systemic vascular resistance
SVT	supraventricular tachycardia
T_3	triiodothyronine
T_4	thyroxine
TB	tuberculosis
TBI	traumatic brain injury
TCA	tricyclic antidepressant
TEE	transesophageal echocardiography
TIPS	transjugular intrahepatic portosystemic shunt
TISS	Therapeutic Intervention Scoring System
TMP	trimethoprim
tPA	tissue-type plasminogen activator
TPN	total parenteral nutrition
TSH	thyroid-stimulating hormone

TTE	transthoracic echocardiography
$\dot{V}$	ventilation
VC	vital capacity
V_d	volume of dead space
$\dot{V}_E$	minute ventilation
V_t	tidal volume
VF	ventricular fibrillation
VT	ventricular tachycardia
WBC	white blood cell
WPW	Wolff–Parkinson–White (syndrome)
ZES	Zollinger–Ellison syndrome

Chapter 1

An approach to critical care

Imre Noth
University of Chicago, Chicago, IL, USA

Introduction

Critical care is an exciting field with diverse and complex challenges. These challenges include identifying pathophysiology in the individual patient, integrating care providers from multiple disciplines, addressing social concerns in the sick or dying patient, to name but a few. As a result of this complexity, care in the intensive care unit (ICU) must be guided by a thoughtful and organized approach.

Providing exemplary care

The first objective is, of course, to provide exemplary care. The intensivist must develop and trust in his or her clinical skills. An effective approach to solving clinical dilemmas in the ICU must involve the development of a clinical hypothesis; the dictum 'don't just do something, stand there' is an invaluable lesson in developing and guiding therapy. Frequently, the level of illness in the ICU can be overwhelming and there is an urge to act quickly, but not necessarily in a directed fashion. This may serve only to further confuse interpretation of the underlying pathophysiologic state. The six steps below are a useful tool for guiding physician behavior in the ICU:

1. Develop and trust one's clinical skills.
2. Formulate clinical hypotheses and test them.
3. Liberate patients from interventions so that treatments do not outnumber diagnoses.
4. Define therapeutic goals and seek the least intervention in achieving each goal.
5. First, do no harm.
6. Organize the critical care team.

Developing and trusting one's clinical skills

It is important initially to take a careful history and physical examination, as it is the nature of the critical care practitioner to act first. By doing this, the disciplined approach to medical practice of developing a differential diagnosis first is inverted. Second, it is important to use all the information at your disposal – this includes the bedside examination, laboratory values, and radiologic findings, in addition to the wealth of information available from monitoring devices. Lastly, it is important to ask oneself what characteristics do not fit, and why they do not fit.

Formulating and testing clinical hypotheses

Testing a therapeutic hypothesis requires knowing the goal of the intervention and titrating a therapy to an endpoint to:

- create a differential diagnosis
- decide on the testable measure
- engage an intervention sufficiently to assess the hypothesis
- reassess.

One example is the common question of whether the patient has an adequate circulating volume. This notion is frequently tested by volume challenge, and physicians early in training are often not aggressive enough in reaching the goal of their intervention. An adult patient presenting in hypovolemic shock cannot be judged to benefit from a small bolus of fluid (eg, 0.25 L 0.9% saline), since the intravascular volume is not likely to be adequately repeated to affect a rise in blood pressure: the testable measure. A bolus should be given in larger initial quantities and assessed frequently to see if the goal of improving blood pressure or (better yet) measures of peripheral organ perfusion are attained.

Ensuring that treatments do not outnumber diagnoses

Daily assessments for continuing or discontinuing the treatment should be conducted, and certain questions should be asked. It is important to ask whether ongoing sedation is necessary. Can the patient undergo a spontaneous breathing trial? If the patient can breathe spontaneously, can they move forward to extubation? Can devices (eg, central lines, pulmonary artery flotation catheters, chest tubes, nasogastric tubes, external or intravenous pacers) be discontinued to facilitate comfort, reduce the need for analgesics and sedatives, and reduce risks such as infection? Are all medications currently employed necessary, and are they likely to interact with each other? These are questions that need to be considered to ensure that the patient receives the best treatment.

Defining therapeutic goals and minimizing intervention

It is difficult to judge the success of a given therapy if treatment goals have not been set. For example, in the case of vasoactive drugs, it is important to recognize that the goal of pharmacologic support is to support the patient until they are adequately resuscitated and to ensure adequate perfusion. There is also a risk–benefit ratio to these goals, and prolonged administration of these drugs at high levels may in fact lead to tissue hypoperfusion. In addition, it is important to set systolic and diastolic blood pressure levels for aggressive resuscitation. Cardiac output (CO) or measures of adequate oxygen delivery (such as mixed venous oxygen saturation) may be better measures of the success of vasoactive support and there is as much opportunity to be aggressive in the discontinuation of these drugs as there is in their initiation.

First, do no harm

Always assess the cost of any intervention or action to be sure that the benefit outweighs the risks. An example is adding positive end-expiratory pressure (PEEP) to help improve oxygenation. While there is often an improvement in oxygenation, there may also be a reduction in preload causing CO to fall and hence oxygen delivery to actually be reduced.

Organizing the critical care team

Fundamentals for team building in the ICU include maintenance of skills, a 'team' attitude, and a structured framework that includes shared rounds and a multidisciplinary management committee. The intensivist is not in charge of the patient as a solo practitioner, but must also take into account the interactions with:

- nurses
- respiratory therapists
- case managers
- physical therapists
- physical plant
- technology
- administrators
- ethicists.

Economics of ICU care

Health-care costs continue to play an ever-increasing role in how physicians engage in medical practice. As resources become more and more limited, physicians must adjust to these changes.

ICU medicine accounted for 1% of the US gross domestic product in the 1990s; this is a disproportionately large portion of health-care resources. In addition, human resources also accounted for the largest fraction of costs, with nursing services representing approximately 40% and physician support approximately 10% of costs. The greatest utilization of resources, however, remains those patients who are predicted to live but die, and those who are predicted to die but live. Despite this there is a substantial benefit to ICU care. Survival rates clearly demonstrate this (eg, 94.6% survive the ICU, 86.5% survive hospitalization, and 55–69% of patients demonstrate survival at 1 year).

Significant cost savings in ICUs can be achieved through improved utilization, decreased length of stay through high-quality care, and use of less costly sites of care delivery when appropriate.

Managing death in the ICU

To many patients survival and return to functionality justify the provision of critical care services; however, it is also true that during the course of ICU management many patients will be identified who are best treated by shifting goals from cure to comfort. This may be the most emotionally demanding and time-consuming activity in the ICU. It is important to recognize that there are many forces at play, from the patient's wishes to the concerns of the family, and finally the sense of investment on the part of the physician.

The patient

The first step is deciding whether the patient is dying. Many physicians are perplexed by the decision to determine medical futility. The factors that help physicians determine when a patient is dying include:
- past medical history
- comorbidities
- number of organ systems in failure
- level of response to therapy of the acute illness.

The family

Once the decision has been made that the patient is dying, the physician is then responsible for communicating this to the patient and family. This will enable the physician to help with decisions to withhold or withdraw life support, and will direct the focus of all concerned to the important process of grieving.

The process
It is important to compassionately address the concerns of the patient, family, physician, and ancillary services. The objective of patient care should be changed from cure to comfort, not eliminated. The change of goals should be undertaken with the same zeal as the aggressive no-nonsense approach when the patient first presents. Figure 1.1 reviews where and how these goals might change.

The experience
The clinician must also be aware that, for some families, it will be their first encounter with death and as such there are several steps that may help to ease the process:

- Ensure that, when withdrawal occurs, the patient is comfortable – this may involve high levels of opiates. The physician should not fear this as the goal has changed and the priority is comfort over life-prolonging measures.
- Remove as many technological connections as possible in an effort to increase human contact.
- Give complete access to family members.
- Ensure that social service or clerical support is available.

Up to 90% of patients who die in ICUs die with the withdrawal of life-sustaining measures; exemplary care helps to ease the transition of treatment to comfort care, and aids in this natural process of life.

ICU quality
Given the high costs of health care and the level of critical illness in the ICU, ensuring quality of care is very important. Quality measures to consider are given in Figure 1.2.

Goals of therapy	
Cure	**Comfort**
Ventilation	Treat pain
Perfusion	Relieve dyspnea
Dialysis	Allay anxiety
Nutrition	Minimize interventions
Treat infection	Family access
Surgery	Support
Differential diagnosis	Grieving

Figure 1.1 Goals of therapy.

Measures of quality in the intensive care unit
Survival rate
Complication rates
Quality of life
Appropriateness of the medical interventions provided
Patient and family satisfaction
Resource utilization
Cost-effectiveness of care

Figure 1.2 Measures of quality in the intensive care unit.

Legal issues

Although many legal issues may arise in the ICU as elsewhere in the hospital, a daily concern is obtaining consent for the many procedures that are required. In order to be considered legally effective, consent to medical treatment must meet three tests:

1. It must be voluntary.
2. The patient must be adequately informed.
3. The obtaining of consent must be by someone with adequate capacity and authority.

It is important to note that physicians rely on family members as surrogate decision-makers for incapacitated patients, even in the absence of a specific statute, advance directive, or court order. In addition, some patients may lack relatives or friends to act as surrogate decision-makers. In such cases, physicians should seek guidance from living wills or other forms of advance directive. Neither a patient nor a family member can demand medical treatment that would be futile, and the physician is not obligated to provide such medical treatment. If the physician and patient or surrogate decision-maker have irreconcilable differences, the physician may help provide alternate care opportunities.

Chapter 2

Analgesia and sedation in the intensive care unit

John Kress
University of Chicago, Chicago, IL, USA

Indications

Indications for analgesia and sedation in the intensive care unit (ICU) are as follows:

- analgesia
- relief of anxiety
- relief of dyspnea
- to facilitate mechanical ventilation
- to diminish autonomic hyperactivity
- to decrease oxygen consumption (VO_2)
- amnesia during neuromuscular blockade.

Available drug types

Several types of sedative available are commonly used in the ICU:

- opioid analgesics
- benzodiazepines
- intravenous anesthetic agents (eg, propofol)
- other sedatives/tranquilizing agents (eg, haloperidol, dexmedetomidine)
- regional anesthetic techniques.

Drug regimens should of course be matched to the particular needs of individual patients; however, generally speaking, no single drug is ideal and what follows is a summary of the advantages and disadvantages of each drug.

Opioid analgesics

Figure 2.1 shows some of the properties of the more common opioid analgesics.

Advantages

- respiratory depression
- analgesia
- cough suppression
- relative cardiovascular stability
- some anxiolysis.

Disadvantages

- inhibition of gastric emptying and gastrointestinal motility
- prolonged duration of action (most agents have a long elimination half-life) and may therefore cause unwanted respiratory depression in patients during liberation from mechanical ventilation
- potential for cardiovascular instability in shock resulting from decreased endogenous catecholamine release

Properties of opioid analgesics

	Fentanyl	Meperidine	Methadone	Morphine
Onset (min)	0.5–1	3–5	10–20	10
Duration (h)	0.5–1	1–4	6–24	4
Metabolism	Hepatic	Hepatic	Hepatic	Hepatic
Elimination	Renal	Renal	Renal	Renal
Anxiolysis	++	++	+	+
Analgesia	++++	++++	++++	++++
Hypnosis	±	±	±	±
Amnesia	No	No	No	No
Seizure threshold	No effect	May lower	No effect	No effect
Dyspnea	++++	++++	++++	++++
CV effects	Venodilate — ↓BP	Venodilate — ↓BP	Venodilate — ↓BP	Venodilate — ↓BP
Respiratory effects	Shift CO_2 response curve to right	Shift CO_2 response curve to right	Shift CO_2 response curve to right	Shift CO_2 response curve to right
Cost	$	$	$	$
Side effects	Nausea, ileus, itching	Seizures	Nausea, ileus, itching	Nausea, ileus, itching, histamine release

All pharmacologic properties are based on a single dose.

Figure 2.1 Properties of opioid analgesics. BP, blood pressure; CV, cardiovascular.

- nausea and vomiting
- ureteric and biliary spasm.

Benzodiazepines

Figure 2.2 shows some of the properties of the more common benzodiazepines.

Advantages

- amnesic
- anxiolytic and hypnotic
- anticonvulsant
- relative cardiovascular stability.

Disadvantages

- no analgesic activity
- unpredictable accumulation and consequent prolonged duration of action
- respiratory depression in spontaneously ventilating patients.

Properties of benzodiazepines

	Diazepam	Lorazepam	Midazolam
Onset (min)	1–3	5	0.5–2
Duration (h)	1–6	6–10	2
Metabolism	Hepatic	Hepatic (less influenced by age and liver disease)	Hepatic
Elimination	Renal (active metabolite)	Renal (no active metabolite)	Renal (active metabolite)
Anxiolysis	++++	++++	++++
Analgesia	±	±	±
Hypnosis	++++	++++	++++
Amnesia	++++	+++	++++
Seizure threshold	+++	++++	+++
Dyspnea	+	+	+
CV effects	Venodilate — $\downarrow$BP	Venodilate — $\downarrow$BP	Venodilate — $\downarrow$BP
Respiratory effects	Shift CO_2 response curve to right	Shift CO_2 response curve to right	Shift CO_2 response curve to right
Cost	$	$	$
Side effects	Occasionally paradoxical agitation	Occasionally paradoxical agitation	Occasionally paradoxical agitation

Figure 2.2 Properties of benzodiazepines. BP, blood pressure; CV, cardiovascular.

Intravenous anesthetic agents

Figure 2.3 shows some of the properties of the more common intravenous anesthetic agents.

Neuromuscular blockade

The routine use of neuromuscular blockade or muscle relaxants to facilitate intubation and ventilation is associated with accelerated muscle atrophy, weaning difficulties, and an increased incidence of nosocomial pneumonia, and consequently it is now discouraged. The remaining indications for prolonged neuromuscular blockade include:

- Refractory hypoxemia in patients with acute hypoxemic respiratory failure (usually severe acute respiratory distress syndrome) – to facilitate ventilation, particularly inverse ratio ventilation and permissive hypercapnia, and to reduce (skeletal muscle) oxygen consumption.

Properties of intravenous anesthetic agents

	Dexmedetomidine	Haloperidol	Propofol
Onset (min)	10	2–5	0.5–5
Duration (h)	2	2	2–8
Metabolism	Hepatic	Hepatic	Hepatic, renal, lungs
Elimination	Renal	Renal	Renal
Anxiolysis	+++	+++	++++
Analgesia	+++	±	No
Hypnosis	++	++	++++
Amnesia	+	No	++++
Seizure threshold	?	No effect	??
Dyspnea	+++	No	+
CV effects	Bradycardia, hypotension	↓BP, QT prolongation (torsades de pointes)	Veno-, arterio-dilation, myocardial suppression
Respiratory effects	No	No	Shift CO_2 response curve to right
Cost	$$$	$	$$
Side effects	Bradycardia, hypotension	Antiemetic, extrapyramidal effects	↑triglycerides, dysrhythmias/CHF, metabolic acidosis

Figure 2.3 **Properties of intravenous anesthetic agents.** BP, blood pressure; CHF, chronic heart failure; CV, cardiovascular.

- Critical intracranial hypertension in whom unwanted motor activity cannot be prevented by sedation alone.
- Tetanus – improves chest wall compliance.

Infusions of short-acting, non-depolarizing relaxants such as vecuronium, atracurium, and *cis*-atracurium are generally used, and should be titrated against response using a monitor of neuromuscular blockade. Prolonged use of an aminosteroid relaxant (eg, vecuronium) is occasionally associated with very prolonged paralysis. Initial recommended doses are:

1. Atracurium 5–10 mg/kg per min (loading dose 0.2 mg/kg)
2. *cis*-Atracurium 1–5 mg/kg per min (loading dose 0.5 mg/kg)
3. Vecuronium 0.8–1.4 mg/kg per min (loading dose 1 mg/kg).

The metabolism of atracurium and *cis*-atracurium is independent of hepatic metabolism and renal excretion, although the excitatory metabolite laudanosine may accumulate in patients with renal failure who are given atracurium. *cis*-Atracurium also has more hemodynamic stability than atracurium. Vecuronium may accumulate in patients with hepatic impairment and is not considered to be a first-line drug in critically ill patients.

Sedation requirements

Sedation should be tailored to the clinical circumstances. For example, the sedative requirements of a patient with critical oxygenation, requiring full mechanical ventilation, are very different from those of a patient with a tracheostomy who is being weaned from ventilation. Several sedation scores are available to help quantify levels of sedation. While the Ramsay Sedation Scale (Figure 2.4) has been employed for the longest period of time, newer scoring systems are being more widely employed in recent years. The Richmond Agitation Sedation Scale (Figure 2.5) is among the most extensively evaluated.

Ramsay Sedation Scale	
1	Anxious, agitated or restless
2	Cooperative, orientated, and tranquil
3	Responds to commands only
4	Asleep, but brisk response to glabellar tap or loud auditory stimulus
5	Asleep, but sluggish response to glabellar tap or loud auditory stimulus
6	No response

Figure 2.4 Ramsay Sedation Scale.

Richmond Agitation Sedation Scale		
+4	Combative	Overtly combative, violent, immediate danger to staff
+3	Very agitated	Pulls or removes tube(s) or catheter(s), aggressive
+2	Agitated	Frequent nonpurposeful movement, fights ventilator
+1	Restless	Anxious but movements not aggressive or vigorous
0	Alert and calm	
−1	Drowsy	Not fully alert, but has sustained awakening (eye opening/eye contact) to *voice* (≥10 seconds)
−2	Light sedation	Briefly awakens with eye contact to *voice* (<10 seconds)
−3	Moderate sedation	Movement or eye opening to *voice* (but no eye contact)
−4	Deep sedation	No response to *voice*, but movement or eye opening to *physical* stimulation
−5	Unarousable	No response to *voice* or *physical* stimulation

Figure 2.5 Richmond Agitation Sedation Scale. Reproduced with permission from Sessler et al. *Am J Respir Crit Care Med* 2002; 166:1338–44.

Complications of sedation in the ICU

Possible complications of sedation in the ICU include:

- cardiovascular instability
- gastric stasis and impaired enteral nutritional support
- reduced mobilization and muscle wasting
- delayed weaning from mechanical ventilation
- nosocomial pneumonia
- drug accumulation and consequent prolonged duration of action
- withdrawal syndromes (typically seen in patients receiving continuous infusions for several days without interruption).

Reduction of sedative requirements in the ICU

All sedatives can accumulate in critically ill patients, leading to a prolonged sedative effect. This may increase the duration of mechanical ventilation, length of stay in the ICU, and length of stay in the hospital, and lead to complications such as ventilator-associated pneumonia. A strategy to reduce drug accumulation should be implemented (eg, a daily interruption of sedative infusions until the patient awakens, or a nursing-directed administration protocol based on a targeted level of sedation).

Daily interruption of sedative infusions is associated with reduced duration of mechanical ventilation and ICU length of stay. Patients subjected to daily sedative interruption are reported to have a reduced long-term psychological maladjustment (eg, post-traumatic stress disorder) after critical illness. This strategy can be used safely in a wide range of patients; even patients at high risk for coronary artery disease can undergo daily sedative interruption without an increased risk of precipitating myocardial ischemia. Other strategies such as regional analgesia to reduce systemic opioid requirements may also be beneficial in selected patients.

Chapter 3

The cardiovascular system

Brian Gehlbach
University of Chicago, Chicago, IL, USA

Pressure monitoring

Indirect and intermittent measurements of vascular pressures are generally considered inadequate in unstable, critically ill patients. Direct measurement involves the connection of a transducer system (with a continuous flushing device) via fluid-filled manometer tubing to a cannula placed in an appropriate vessel. The advantages of this include:

- continuous information on arterial and venous pressures
- information is available from waveform analysis
- (arterial) blood sampling.

There are potential sources of error in pressure measurement, namely zero errors and kinks or clots in the manometer tube.

Zero errors include inaccurate zeroing of the transducer or imprecise placement of the transducer (this is particularly important in venous pressure measurement, when absolute pressure is small). Kinks, clots, or bubbles in the manometer tubing can lead to damping or resonance. Damping refers to flattening of the pressure trace, underestimating systolic and overestimating diastolic pressures; the mean is accurate. Resonance refers to an overshoot of pressure waveform due to resonant oscillations within the measuring system. It overestimates systolic and underestimates diastolic pressure; the mean is accurate.

Arterial pressure monitoring

The radial, ulnar, femoral, and dorsalis pedis arteries are commonly used for arterial pressure monitoring. End-arteries such as the brachial artery should be avoided, if possible. Complications include:

- hemorrhage from puncture sites or open taps (which can be severe if unrecognized)

- thrombosis
- drug injection with subsequent ischemia
- infection
- nerve injury.

Central venous catheterization

Figures 3.1–3.2 show the main sites for insertion of central venous catheters, and the complications associated with this, respectively.

Sites for insertion of central venous catheters	
Basilic vein (antecubital fossa)	Avoids damage to structures of thoracic inlet, neck Maneuvering past clavipectoral fascia may be difficult, but correct placement in up to 90% of patients in experienced hands Risk of damage to brachial artery and median nerve Thrombophlebitis is common Traditionally performed using single-lumen 'long lines'
External jugular vein	May be difficult to find Potentially less damaging to neck structures and lung than internal jugular May be awkward to pass guidewire into SVC because of tortuous route Useful for temporary emergency access
Femoral vein	'Long lines' required to allow CVP measurement Useful when clotting is deranged or when patient will not tolerate head-down position Convenient site for large-bore devices (eg, dialysis catheters) Higher risk for infection, thrombosis
Internal jugular vein	Reliable access to SVC and right atrium Risk of damage to neck structures (hematoma from punctured carotid artery can cause life-threatening airway obstruction) Lower risk of pneumothorax than subclavian vein Less comfortable for patient
Subclavian vein	Popular choice with the inexperienced Higher rate of pneumothorax (up to 20%) Bleeding from punctured subclavian artery difficult to control Generally comfortable for patients (although awkward for treatment of shoulder contractures in neurologic/neurosurgical patients) Probably lowest infection rate Suitable for tunneling

Figure 3.1 Sites for insertion of central venous catheters. CVP, central venous pressure; SVC, superior vena cava.

Complications of central venous catheter insertion	
Catheter residence	**Venous puncture**
Catheter-related sepsis	Arterial puncture
Thrombosis (venous and cardiac)	Pneumothorax
Venous stenosis	Air embolism (minimized by head-down position)
Phlebitis	
Endocarditis	Damage to larynx, thyroid, thoracic duct, esophagus, endotracheal tube, brachial plexus, recurrent laryngeal nerve
Erosion through SVC/right atrium	
Dysrhythmias	
Ectopic placement and delivery of fluid (eg, into pleural cavity)	

Figure 3.2 Complications of central venous catheter insertion. SVC, superior vena cava.

Indications

Indications for central venous catheterization include:
- monitoring central venous pressure (CVP)
- infusion of irritant solutions
- infusion of vasoactive drugs
- inadequate peripheral venous access
- long-term venous access (home total parenteral nutrition [TPN], cystic fibrosis, chemotherapy)
- aspiration of air/amniotic fluid (following embolism)
- access to central circulation (endocardial pacing, hemodialysis, pulmonary artery catheterization).

Measurement of central venous pressure

The aim is to measure the pressure of blood within the intrathoracic portion of the superior/inferior vena cava. Clinically, this is usually done by an externally placed measuring device, the pressure being transmitted to it by a column of fluid within a centrally placed catheter (Figure 3.3). The pressure is measured relative to a reference point; traditionally, the intersection of the midaxillary line and the fourth intercostal space with the patient in the supine position. Values will be lower if patients are sitting up or erect.

Interpretation of central venous pressure measurements

The ventricular volume at end-diastole is an important determinant of stroke volume and cardiac output. CVP is used as an indirect estimate of right ventricular end-diastolic volume (RVEDV) as shown in Figure 3.4.

Methods of central venous pressure measurement

Fluid-filled U-tube manometer	Piezoelectric transducer
Pressure expressed as cmH_2O ($1\ cmH_2O = 0.76\ mmHg$)	Pressure expressed as mmHg ($1\ mmHg = 1.3\ cmH_2O$)
Requires no expensive monitoring or consumables	Requires monitoring hardware
Discrete rather than continuous measurement	Real-time continuous measurement
No waveform	Waveform available
Prone to zero errors	Prone to zero errors
Labor intensive	Consumable costs
Risk of inadvertent air embolism	

Figure 3.3 Methods of central venous pressure measurement.

The relationship between CVP and left ventricular end-diastolic volume (LVEDV) is even more indirect. Trends are more important than absolute values, particularly dynamic responses to fluid therapy or inotropes (Figure 3.5).

Pulmonary artery catheterization

Pulmonary artery catheters (PACs) are multilumen catheters, 80–120 cm, introduced into the pulmonary artery through a central (systemic) vein. Lumina opening at 25–30 cm from the tip allow measurement of CVP and central delivery of drugs, while the distal lumen (pulmonary) opens at the tip. Figure 3.6 shows the information that is potentially obtainable using this type of catheter.

Insertion

The catheter is passed through a specifically designed introducer sited in a central vein (preferably the right internal jugular or left subclavian, but any central vein is acceptable, as are the femoral and basilic veins). Inflation of the balloon at the tip of the catheter once it is in the central circulation facilitates correct placement, which is followed by monitoring the pressure waveforms measured at the tip of the catheter as it is introduced. Some of the complications associated with using pulmonary artery catheters are given in Figure 3.7.

Pulmonary artery wedge pressure (PAWP)

Inflation of the balloon at the tip of a correctly positioned PAC seals the surrounding artery and so creates a continuous, stationary column of blood between the tip of the catheter and the left atrium. This 'wedge' pressure is a measure

Relationship between CVP and RVEDV

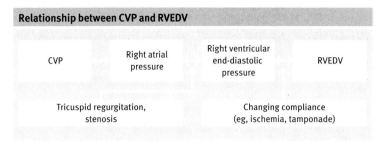

Figure 3.4 Relationship between CVP and RVEDV. CVP, central venous pressure; RVEDV, right ventricular end-diastolic volume.

Hemodynamic response to fluid challenges

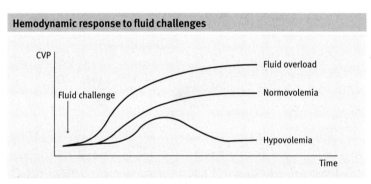

Figure 3.5 Hemodynamic response to fluid challenges. CVP, central venous pressure.

Data derived from pulmonary artery catheters

Directly measured	Pulmonary artery pressure (systolic, mean, diastolic)
	Pulmonary artery wedge pressure
	CVP
	Blood temperature
	Mixed venous oxygen saturation/content
Estimated	Cardiac output (discrete or continuous)
Derived (requiring other information:	Cardiac index
BP, heart rate, CVP, etc.)	Systemic and pulmonary vascular resistance
	Stroke volume
	Cardiac work
	Oxygen delivery and consumption variables

Figure 3.6 Data derived from pulmonary artery catheters. BP, blood pressure; CVP, central venous pressure.

Complications of using pulmonary artery catheters

Catheterization	Dysrhythmias (which can be severe and may persist after withdrawal)
	RBBB, which may precipitate complete heart block in a patient with existing LBBB
	Catheter knotting
	Atrial and ventricular perforation
	Valvular injury
Catheter residence	Pulmonary artery rupture (particularly in patients with pulmonary hypertension)
	Sepsis
	Thrombophlebitis
	Venous thrombosis
	Pulmonary infarction
	Mural thrombus
	Valvular vegetations/endocarditis
	Death
Derived (requiring other information:	Cardiac index
BP, heart rate, CVP, etc.)	Systemic and pulmonary vascular resistance
	Stroke volume
	Cardiac work
	Oxygen delivery and consumption variables

Figure 3.7 Complications of using pulmonary artery catheters. LBBB, left bundle-branch block; RBBB, right bundle-branch block.

of the filling pressure of the left ventricle, and indirectly of LVEDV. Sources of error are shown in Figure 3.8.

Measuring cardiac output by thermodilution using a PAC

A known volume of cold injectate is delivered into the CVP lumen of a PAC. The time integral of the temperature change measured by a thermistor at the tip of the pulmonary artery flotation catheter (PAFC) is used to calculate the cardiac output according to the Stewart–Hamilton equation thus:

$$\dot{Q} = \frac{[1.08 \times k \times V] \times (T_b - T_i)}{m\delta T \times t}$$

where k = catheter constant; T_b = blood temperature; V = volume of injectate; T_i = injectate temperature; $m\delta T$ = mean temperature change; $\dot{Q}$ = cardiac output; t = duration of temperature change.

Sources of error in PAWP measurement

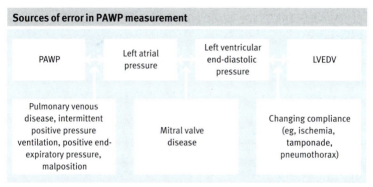

Figure 3.8 Sources of error in PAWP measurement. LVEDV, left ventricular end-diastolic volume; PAWP, pulmonary artery wedge pressure.

Hemodynamic variables derived from a PAC

These indices (ie, variables expressed per unit body surface area) depend critically upon estimates of height and weight, and so may be liable to considerable error. Correction factors, omitted from the formulae for the sake of clarity, are often required to relate normal values to commonly used units of pressure, length, time, etc. As with CVP monitoring, responses to therapy are more important than absolute values.

Indications for placement of a PAC

Figure 3.9 shows some of the variables that can be derived from a PAC; however, studies that have failed to demonstrate an improved outcome in critical patients have cast doubt on the clinical value of PACs. Nevertheless, traditional indications include the following:

- Hemodynamic instability unresponsive to inotropic therapy/fluid therapy guided by CVP measurement – proponents of PAC placement argue that inotropes may be more rationally used if cardiac output and PAWP have been measured.
- Conditions in which CVP is a poor guide to LVEDV – left ventricular dysfunction valvular heart disease, pulmonary hypertension, extracardiac causes of diastolic dysfunction (eg, tense ascites).
- Severe sepsis/systemic inflammatory response syndrome (SIRS).
- Acute renal failure, particularly when combined with respiratory and hemodynamic failure.
- Acute respiratory distress syndrome, particularly to guide fluid therapy.

Variables derived from a pulmonary artery catheter

Parameter	Formula	Normal values
Cardiac index	CO/BSA	3–4 L/min per m²
Pulmonary vascular resistance index	[(MPAP – PAWP) × 80]/CI	200–400 dyn s m²/cm⁵
Stroke volume	CO/HR	55–100 mL
Stroke index	CO/(HR × BSA)	35–70 mL/m²
Systemic vascular resistance index	[(MPAP – CVP) × 80]/CI	1,600–2,400 dyn s m²/cm⁵

Figure 3.9 Variables derived from a pulmonary artery catheter. BSA, body surface area; CI, cardiac index; CO, cardiac output; CVP, central venous pressure; HR, heart rate; MAP, mean arterial pressure; MPAP, mean pulmonary artery pressure; PAWP, pulmonary artery wedge pressure.

- Some perioperative situations – high-risk surgery, myocardial infarction within the previous 6 months, risk of air embolism (eg, neurosurgery in sitting position).

To date, the use of PAC monitoring has not been shown to confer a clinical benefit in any of these settings.

Noninvasive cardiovascular monitoring

Doppler flow measurements

Blood flow velocities can be calculated by measuring the frequency shift of an incident ultrasonic wave (2–20 MHz), taking into account the angle of incidence of the sound beam. The product of velocity and cross-sectional area gives flow. Modes are outlined below.

Suprasternal monitoring

The transcutaneous measurement of blood velocity in the ascending aorta/ arch, can be done with the incident wave being directed toward the aortic arch. A graphical display of velocity versus time confirms the correct orientation. Derivation of the aortic cross-sectional area, from nomograms, allows cardiac output (CO) to be calculated. Accuracy is limited by variation in angles of incidence and nonuniformity of flow velocities across the vessel.

Esophageal Doppler monitoring (EDM)

A probe is placed in the distal third of the esophagus, which measures blood velocity in the descending aorta. A graphical display of velocity versus time confirms the correct orientation. Errors due to variations in angles of incidence or nonuniform flow are less significant. The aortic cross-sectional area is derived from nomograms, and CO is calculated assuming that 70% of CO goes down the descending aorta. There is a good correlation with other estimates of CO, and an analysis of velocity-time profile gives qualitative information on inotropic state and filling.

Thoracic electrical bioimpedance
Thoracic electrical bioimpedance estimates CO from the changes in thoracic cavity electrical conductivity, which result from the changing blood volume, during the cardiac cycle. It is a totally noninvasive technique that is useful as a trend monitor, but has limited absolute accuracy.

Echocardiography
Uses of two-dimensional echocardiography in the ICU include the following:
- Diagnosis of valvular abnormalities – stenosis, incompetence, vegetations, papillary muscle rupture
- Diagnosis of structural abnormalities – congenital defects, acquired septal defects, myocardial hypertrophy, dilation, regional wall-motion abnormalities, suggesting ischemia, ventricular aneurysms, mural thrombi, overall ventricular function, with assessment of ejection fraction
- Assessment of ventricular filling in guiding fluid therapy
- Diagnosis of pericardial effusions/tamponade
- Guide to pericardial drainage

Two techniques of echocardiography are described below.

Transthoracic echocardiography
Transthoracic echocardiography (TTE) is noninvasive, employing parasternal, apical, subcostal, and suprasternal windows. There is access to most areas of the heart, but views of the mitral valve, aorta, and atria may be limited. Examination may be suboptimal in patients with obesity, emphysema, other hyperinflation states, and those who are mechanically ventilated.

Transesophageal echocardiography
In transesophageal echocardiography (TEE) an acoustic transducer is mounted at the tip of a modified endoscope, with views taken through the esophagus and stomach. It requires sedation/topical anesthesia. This is a useful option among patients in the ICU when TTE fails, and is superior to TTE in diagnosing left atrial disease (eg, thrombus, endocarditis). It is becoming a standard diagnostic tool for aortic dissection. Intraoperative use also permits a real-time assessment of left ventricular performance.

Inotropic support

Inotropes/vasopressors

A wide range of inotropes and vasopressors is available to help support CO or blood pressure (BP). They should be used in conjunction with measures to optimize ventricular filling as guided by clinical assessment and measurement of CVP/PAWP. Inotropes increase contractility and hence CO, but their effect on blood pressure is variable depending upon the effect on vascular resistance. Inotropes that vasodilate and vasoconstrict are known as inodilators and ino-constrictors, respectively. Vasoconstrictors should always increase blood pressure, but may have a variable effect on CO. Many of these drugs have the potential to cause myocardial ischemia due to increases in cardiac workload, tachy-carrhythmias, etc, and thus as electrocardiogram (EKG) and (preferably direct) arterial pressure monitoring are mandatory during their use. Vasoconstrictor drugs must be given into a central vein.

Phosphodiesterase inhibitors

Phosphodiesterase inhibitors are inodilators that act by inhibiting the break-down of cAMP (cyclic adenosine 3':5'-monophosphate) in cardiac and vascular smooth muscle. They may be of benefit in patients with cardiogenic shock or heart failure complicated by pulmonary hypertension, such as mitral valve disease, but tachydysrhythmias limit their use (Figure 3.10).

Intravenous phosphodiesterase inhibitor regimen		
Drug	Loading dose	Infusion
Milrinone	50 µg/kg	0.3–0.75 µg/kg per min

Figure 3.10 Intravenous phosphodiesterase inhibitor regimen.

Catecholamines

Catecholamines are active at adrenergic and dopaminergic receptors. Their varied clinical effects are explained by their differing activities at the various adrenergic and dopaminergic receptors (Figures 3.11 and 3.12).

Nonpharmacologic circulatory support

Intra-aortic balloon counterpulsation

A balloon-tipped catheter is surgically introduced into the thoracic aorta through the femoral artery. Inflation of the balloon with 50 mL CO_2 or helium during diastole increases intra-aortic pressure, and augments coronary per-

Effects mediated by adrenoceptor subtypes		
Receptor	**Location**	**Activity**
α_1	Blood vessels	Vasoconstriction
	Myocardium	Inotropy
	Bronchi	Bronchoconstriction
	Uterus	Contraction
	Bladder sphincter	Contraction
	Gastrointestinal tract	
	Shincter	Contraction
	Nonsphincter	Relaxation
	Liver	Glycogenolysis
β_1	Fat	Lipolysis
	Myocardium	Inotropy, chronotropy
β_2	Blood vessels	Vasodilation
	Myocardium	Inotropy, chronotropy
	Bronchi	Bronchodilation
	Uterus	Relaxation
	Bladder detrusor	Relaxation
	Skeletal muscle	Tremor
	Liver	Glycogenolysis

Figure 3.11 Effects mediated by adrenoceptor subtypes.

fusion pressure and distal aortic flow. Rapid deflation during systole reduces left ventricular pressure loading. The overall effect is to increase myocardial perfusion and improve CO by up to 50%. Full anticoagulation is required, and complications from arteriotomy are not uncommon. It should be used only when an improvement in cardiac performance is anticipated (eg, following cardiopulmonary bypass) or as a bridge to transplantation.

Left ventricular assist devices
A variety of 'prosthetic ventricles' is available designed for more long-term use than intra-aortic balloon pumping. Blood is taken from the venous system of the left ventricle and pumped into the aorta. The use of these devices is developmental and restricted to a few specialized units.

Hemodynamic profile of shock states
Figure 3.13 shows the hemodynamic profile associated with various shock states.

Clinical effects of catecholamines at various receptors

Drug	α_1	β_1	β_2	DA_1	Dose (μg/kg per min)	Comments
Dobutamine	0	+++	++	0	2.5–10	Inodilator, useful in low output/high SVR states such as cardiogenic shock. Also useful for the cardiac dysfunction often seen in sepsis/SIRS
Dopamine						
Low dose	0			+++	1–4	Dose-dependent effects. Increased splanchnic/renal blood flow and diuretic effect at low doses, but no evidence for renal protective activity
Medium dose		+	+	+++	5–10	
High dose	+	+	+	+++	>10	May inhibit gastric emptying
Dopexamine	0	0	+++	++	0.5–6	Inodilator licensed for treatment of heart failure following cardiac surgery. Increases hepatosplanchnic blood flow, and may ameliorate gut ischemia in SIRS
Epinephrine	+ to +++	+++	++	0	0.01–0.2	High β-adrenoceptor activity, increasing cardiac output. Vasodilation may be seen at low doses, vasoconstriction at higher doses
Isoproterenol	0	+++	+++	0	0.01–0.2	Potent β agonist, hence risk of tachydysrhythmias. Generally reserved for emergency treatment of bradydysrhythmias and AV block prior to pacing. Now replaced by salbutamol in the management of acute severe asthma
Norepinephrine	+++	+	0	0	0.01–0.2	Inoconstrictor. Very useful in high output/low SVR states such as severe SIRS/sepsis. Inotropic effect via myocardial α-receptors and β activity. May cause reflex bradycardia. Risk of peripheral and splanchnic ischemia
Phenylephrine	+++	0	0	0	0.2–1	Pure vasoconstrictor. Useful alternative to norepinephrine (eg, if arrhythmias are a problem)
Salbutamol	0	+	+++	0	0.1–1	Useful in treatment of acute severe asthma

Figure 3.12 Clinical effects of catecholamines at various receptors. AV, aortic valve; DA, dopamine; SIRS, systemic inflammatory response syndrome; SVR, systemic vascular resistance.

Hemodynamic profile of various shock states

Variable	Cardiac failure	Cardiogenic shock	Septic shock	Hypovolemia	Pulmonary embolism
BP	Variable	↓	↓	N/↓	N/↓
CO	N/↓	↓	Variable	N/↓	N/↓
CVP	N/↑	↑	Variable	N/↓	N/↑
PAP	Variable	Variable	N/↓	N/↓	N/↑
PAWP	N/↑	↑	Variable	N/↓	N/↓
PVR	N/↑	N/↑	N/↑	Variable	N/↑
SV	N/↓	N/↓	Variable	N/↓	N/↓
SVR	N/↑	N/↑	↓	N/↑	N/↑

Figure 3.13 Hemodynamic profile of various shock states. BP, blood pressure; CO, cardiac output; CVP, central venous pressure; N, normal; PAP, pulmonary artery pressure; PAWP, pulmonary artery wedge pressure; PVR, peripheral vascular resistance; SV, stroke volume; SVR, systemic vascular resistance.

Hypertension and hypotensive agents

Hypertension is not uncommon in critically ill patients and may worsen myocardial ischemia and increase oxygen requirements. Causes such as inadequate sedation or analgesia and hypercapnia should be treated in an appropriate fashion. Injudicious use of hypotensive drugs reduces perfusion pressure (eg, kidney, brain, myocardium) and may lead to organ dysfunction.

Adrenergic blocking drugs

All β blockers, even those with apparent cardioselectivity ($\beta_1 > \beta_2$), should be avoided in patients with asthma and in those with cardiac conduction defects as they may precipitate heart failure (Figure 3.14).

Malignant hypertension

This is severe progressive hypertension, with a diastolic pressure of 100 mmHg, and is associated with the following symptoms:
- proteinuric renal failure
- encephalopathy (visual disturbance, altered level of consciousness, seizures, intracerebral hemorrhage)
- grade IV retinal changes (papilledema, fundal hemorrhage)
- left ventricular failure.

Treatment

The upper pressure limit for autoregulation of organ perfusion will be correspondingly higher, so precipitate reductions in pressure may induce cerebral,

Adrenergic blocking drugs

Drug	α_1	β_1	β_2	Dose	Comments
Atenolol	0	+++	+	Orally: 50 mg daily IV bolus: 2.5 mg at 1 mg/min, repeated at 5 min intervals to maximum of 10 mg IV infusion: 150 µg/kg over 20 min repeated every 12 h	Oral administration may be useful in convalescent period IV formulation is used to treat some tachydysrhythmias Bradycardias are common
Esmolol	0	+++	+	Supraventricular tachycardia: 500 µg/kg over 2 min followed by infusion of 50–200 µg/kg per min. Hypertension: 80 mg over 15–30 s followed by infusion of 150–300 µg/kg per min	Short half-life (9 min) due to metabolism by plasma esterases
Labetalol	+++	++	++	Bolus: up to 50 mg over 1 min, repeated every 5 min to a maximum of 200 mg. Infusion: 5–40 µg/kg per min	May cause bronchospasm Significant bradycardia is unusual
Phenoxybenzamine	+++	0	0	10 mg orally, increasing to 1–2 mg/kg in two divided doses	Long-acting non-competitive α blocker, used in combination with β blocker in management of pheochromocytoma; postural hypotension common
Phentolamine	+++	0	0	Bolus: 0.5–5 mg Infusion: 0.5–20 µg/kg per min	Short-acting competitive α blocker given intravenously; postural hypotension common
Propranolol	0	+++	+++	1 mg i.v., repeated to a maximum of 10 mg	Non-selective β blocker useful in emergency treatment of thyrotoxicosis

Figure 3.14 Adrenergic blocking drugs. IV, intravenous.

myocardial, or renal ischemia. Airway management as appropriate in patients with altered conscious levels. Benzodiazepines can be used to control seizures. Hypotensive therapy can also be used; oral treatment if possible, for example, with β blockers, calcium channel blockers, and angiotensin-converting enzyme inhibitors (caution with renal impairment). Intravenous therapy can be administered using labetalol, hydralazine, and sodium nitroprusside (beware cyanide toxicity).

Vasodilators

See Figure 3.15 on page 30.

Arrhythmias and their treatment

Arrythmias are common in the seriously ill and can be caused by:

- pre-existing myocardial disease
- thoracic, cardiac surgery/trauma
- homeostatic disturbances (eg, SIRS, hypokalemia, hyperkalemia, hypomagnesemia, acidosis, hypoxia, hypovolemia, hypo- and hyperthermia)
- iatrogenic factors – drugs (particularly any agent with chronotropic properties, eg, catecholamines, phosphodiesterase inhibitors), catheters within the endocardium (particularly PACs).

Figure 3.16 shows antiarryhthmic drugs classified using the Vaughan–Williams classification system, which categorizes each drug according to the primary mechanism of its antiarrhythmic effect. Figure 3.17 shows the most commonly used antiarrhythmic drugs used in the treatment of arrhythmias.

Supraventricular arrhythmias
Atrial fibrillation

Atrial fibrillation is common in critically ill patients; the EKG shows loss of P-wave with complete irregularity of QRS complexes; it is poorly tolerated when the ventricular response is high due to reduction in ventricular filling time.

Treatment involves synchronized direct current (DC) cardioversion, but this is usually unsuccessful unless a reversible cause is identified and treated. Digoxin controls heart rate only when sympathetic tone is not high; it does not cardiovert. Amiodarone controls rate and cardioverts. Occasionally other drugs (eg, flecainide) can be used.

Supraventricular tachycardia

Supraventricular tachycardia (SVT) includes atrial flutter, junctional tachycardia, and atrial tachycardia.

Vasodilating agents

Drug	Dose	Comments
Angiotensin-converting enzyme inhibitors		
Captopril	Oral/nasogastric: 12.5 mg daily initially, building up to 25–50 mg every 8 h if treatment is tolerated	Useful in treating associated heart failure in patients struggling to wean from mechanical ventilation. Must be introduced with caution, particularly in patients with renal impairment. Also useful in treatment of hypertension
Enalapril	Oral/nasogastric: 2.5–5 mg initially, building up to 20 mg (heart failure) to 40 mg (severe hypertension)	
Calcium channel blockers		
Clevidipine	1–2 mg i.v. per h followed by 4–6 mg i.v. per h	Ultra short-acting; suitable for use in patients with end-organ damage
Nifedipine	10–20 mg sublingually/intranasally every 8 h	Arterial dilation; useful in hypertensive patients in convalescent phase of critical care unable to take oral medication
Nimodipine	Oral: 60 mg every 4 h IV infusion: 1–2 mg/h	Used in spontaneous and traumatic subarachnoid hemorrhage; variable systemic effects
Verapamil	5–10 mg by slow IV bolus	Useful in management of supraventricular arrhythmias; often complicated by severe hypotension. Avoid in patients treated with β blockers due to risk of asystole
Fenoldopam		
	0.1 μg/kg per min, increase in increments of 0.05–0.2 μg/kg i.v.	A selective postsynaptic dopamine agonist that reduces peripheral vascular resistance and enhances renal function
Hydralazine		
	Bolus: 5–10 mg over 20 min, repeated after 20–30 min if necessary Infusion: 1–4 μg/kg per min	Direct arterial dilation; tachycardia may be a problem
Nitrates		
Glyceryl trinitrate	0.25–5 mg/kg per min	Venous dilation; may improve myocardial perfusion and prevent tissue hypoxia during vasoconstrictor therapy. Cause cerebral vasodilation (hence headache) and tachycardia. Tachyphylaxis often seen
Isosorbide dinitrate	0.5–2.5 mg/kg per min	
Sodium nitroprusside		
	Malignant hypertension: 0.25–5 μg/kg per min Induced hypertension: 0.25–1.5 μg/kg per min	Direct arterial and venous dilation. Short half-life allows precise control of arterial pressure. Cyanide toxicity is possible if dose exceeds 8 μg/kg per min (suspect if metabolic acidosis, unexplained tachycardia or arrhythmias, sweating, hyperventilation) Treatment is one of the following: (1) dicobalt edetate 300 mg over 1 min followed by 50 mL 50% glucose or (2) sodium nitrite 300 mg (10 mL of 3% solution) over 3 min followed by 12.5 g sodium thiosulfate (25 mL 50% solution) over 10 min

Figure 3.15 Vasodilating agents.

Vaughan–Williams classification of antiarrhythmic agents

Class	Mechanism(s) of action	Examples
I	Blockade of voltage-sensitive sodium channels, reducing excitability	
Ia	Moderate prolongation of conduction and repolarization	Quinidine, disopyramide, procainamide
Ib	Minimal effect on conduction and repolarization	Lidocaine, phenytoin, tocainide, mexilitine
Ic	Marked prolongation of conduction	Flecainide, propafenone, propranolol, timolol
II	β-Adrenergic blockade, reducing the effect of sympathetic stimulation on the heart	Metoprolol
III	Blockade of repolarizing potassium channel(s), prolongation of refractory period	*d*-Sotalol (pure class III) *dl*-Sotalol, amiodarone
IV	Calcium channel blockers	Diltiazem, verapamil, nifedipine

Figure 3.16 Vaughan–Williams classification of antiarrhythmic agents.

Atrial flutter shows 'saw-tooth' waves on EKG at frequency 300/min. It is associated with a ventricular rate of up to 300/min. Variable ratios of atrioventricular (AV) block give lower ventricular responses (eg, 2:1 block giving rate of 150/min).

Junctional tachycardia is a classic SVT. The EKG shows narrow complex tachycardia at 150–280/min; retrograde atrial conduction of focus may produce abnormal P-waves hidden within the QRS complex. AV or bundle-branch block may occur at higher rates.

Atrial tachycardia involves a narrow complex tachycardia with abnormal P-wave.

Treatment involves synchronized DC cardioversion, particularly if the patient is hemodynamically compromised. Induction of brief AV block allows identification of an underlying atrial rhythm, differentiates SVT with bundle-branch block from ventricular tachycardia, and may terminate arrhythmia. Supraventricular tachycardia can be induced with carotid sinus massage or adenosine (3 mg increasing to 6 mg increasing to 12 mg). Verapamil can also be used, but is best avoided in patients who have received β blockers, due to risk of bradyarrhythmias or asystole. In refractory cases consider using antiarrhythmics, AV blocking drugs (eg, calcium channel blockers, β blockers), and amiodarone.

Commonly used antiarrhythmic agents

Drug	Actions and indications	Dose and administration	Cautions and side effects
Adenosine	Slows sinus rate and prolongs conduction through AV node by acting on specific cardiac adenosine receptors. Drug of choice for AV nodal and AV re-entry tachycardias (eg, WPW syndrome). Also allows (broad-complex) supraventricular tachycardias to be distinguished from ventricular tachycardia	3–6 mg by rapid bolus injection, followed by saline flush to ensure central delivery. Follow with 12 mg and then 18 mg if necessary. Heart transplant recipients are sensitive to adenosine, and should always receive an initial dose of 3 mg. In patients receiving dipyridamole, initial dose should be reduced to 0.5–1 mg	Very short half-life (12–15 s) is a major advantage. Effects are antagonised by theophyllines and enhanced by dipyridamole. May cause transient bronchospasm, and should be avoided in people with asthma. Patients may experience temporary flushing, dyspnea, and chest pain
Amiodarone	Of considerable value in treatment of atrial and ventricular tachyarrhythmias in the critical care setting. Prolongs action potential duration and increases refractory period in all cardiac tissues	300 mg in 100 mL 5% dextrose over 1 h, followed by 900 mg over 23 h, then 600 mg/day for 7 days, then 100–400 mg/day. Convert to oral administration wherever possible. IV doses should be administered via central catheter	Long half-life (50 days). Little negative inotropic action. Side effects common: photosensitivity, corneal deposits, dry cough, hypo- and hyperthyroidism, pulmonary and retroperitoneal fibrosis, peripheral neuropathy, altered liver function tests. Therapeutic level 1–2.5 µg/mL. Dosages of warfarin and digoxin should be halved
Bretyllium	Used in the management of refractory ventricular arrhythmias during resuscitation	5 mg/kg over 15–20 min, followed by 0.5–2 mg/min by continuous infusion	Initial pressor response (believed to be the result of norepinephrine release) is followed by severe postural hypotension

Figure 3.17 Commonly used antiarrhythmic agents. AV, atrioventricular; AF, atrial fibrillation; CNS, central nervous system; EKG, electrocardiogram; IV, intravenous; LV, left ventricular; WPW, Wolff–Parkinson–White (syndrome).

Commonly used antiarrhythmic agents (continued)

Drug	Description	Dose	Notes
Digoxin	Inhibits Na^+/K^+ ATPase, increasing intracellular [Ca^{2+}] and exerting positive inotropic effect. Other actions: prolongation of AV nodal conduction and refractory period, increased automaticity, and vagotonic effect. Indicated in treatment of congestive cardiac failure with AF, in control of chronic AF and management of paroxysmal AF (although agents such as amiodarone that reduce the incidence of paroxysmal episodes are first-line therapy)	IV: 250–500 mg over 10–20 min, repeated over 4–8 h to a maximum of 1 mg. IV loading is associated with very high plasma levels transiently. Oral: 1–1.5 mg over 24 h in two to three divided doses, followed by 62.5–500 mg daily according to renal function	Avoid in secondary or tertiary heart block, WPW syndrome, hypertrophic obstructive cardiomyopathy, recurrent ventricular arrhythmias, before cardioversion. Therapeutic plasma levels 0.8–2 ng/mL (1–2.5 nmol/L). Biological activity increased by hypokalemia, hypercalcemia, hypomagnesemia, hypothyroidism. Plasma elimination half-life 30 h, determined by renal function. Features of toxicity: anorexia, nausea, sinus bradycardia, AV block, ventricular arrhythmias. Digoxin overdose now treated with digoxin antibody fragment
Disopyramide	Class Ia: prolongs action potential and produces dose-dependent slowing of conduction through His–Purkinje system. Has significant anticholinergic effects. Used to treat ventricular and supraventricular tachycardias, although not a first-line drug in either	2 mg/kg i.v. over 5 min to a maximum of 150 mg, followed by 400 mg/kg per h by IV infusion or 200 mg every 8 h by mouth for 24 h	Significant negative inotropic properties. Avoid in secondary or tertiary heart block, heart failure, sinus node dysfunction. Anticholinergic side effects (eg, dry mouth, blurred vision, urinary hesitancy/retention, constipation) most common. Excreted renally (half-life 8–9 h). Therapeutic plasma levels 2–5 µg/mL
Flecainide	Class Ic: slows conduction in all cardiac tissues. Potentially useful in supraventricular, AV nodal, and AV re-entry tachycardias, although other agents (adenosine, verapamil) are more popular in the acute setting. May also have a role in life-threatening ventricular arrhythmias	IV: 2 mg/kg over 10–15 min to maximum of 150 mg, with continuous EKG monitoring. Can be followed by infusion of 1.5 mg/kg per h for 1 h, then 0.1–0.25 mg/kg per h for 24 h. Maximum IV dose is 600 mg. Oral: 50–200 mg every 12 h	Negatively inotrope, may induce refractory ventricular arrhythmias. Increases mortality in patients with acute myocardial infarction. Contraindicated in heart failure, secondary and tertiary heart block, sinoatrial disease and pacemakers (pacing threshold may rise). Eliminated by hepatic metabolism. Therapeutic plasma level 0.2–1 µg/mL

Figure 3.17 Continued. AF, atrial fibrillation; ATPase, adenosine triphosphatase; AV, atrioventricular; Ca, calcium; EKG, echocardiogram; IV, intravenous; K, potassium; Na, sodium; WPW, Wolff–Parkinson–White (syndrome).

Commonly used antiarrhythmic agents (continued)

Lidocaine	Class Ib: first-line therapy in acute ventricular tachyarrhythmias. Shortens action potential by blocking Na⁺ channels. No effect on sinus rate, sinoatrial node function, or conduction through His–Purkinje system. Of no value in treatment of supraventricular arrhythmias	Must be given intravenously. Typical dosage schedule is 1.5–2 mg/kg as bolus over 5 min, with a further 1 mg/kg if ineffective, followed by 4 mg/min for 1 h, then 2 mg/min for 2 h and 1 mg/min. Omit 4 mg/min stage in low-output states	Rapidly metabolized in liver (half-life 1–2 h). Reduce dose by 30–50% in liver or heart failure. Therapeutic plasma levels 1.5–6 µg/mL. Signs of CNS toxicity include anxiety, tremor, metallic taste, circumoral paresthesia, convulsions, and coma
Magnesium	Mg²⁺ is essential cofactor for Na⁺/K⁺ ATPase; deficiency causes intracellular hypokalemia that cannot be corrected with K⁺ supplements alone, accounting for arrhythmogenic consequences. Plasma levels do not reflect intracellular concentration. Indicated in treatment of life-threatening ventricular arrhythmias, eg, torsades de pointes, those associated with hypokalemia, and digoxin toxicity	IV: 8 mmol over 10–15 min, repeated if necessary	Side effects are features of hypermagnesemia: flushing, hypotension, muscle weakness, respiratory depression
Verapamil	Class IV, prolonging conduction through and increasing refractory period of AV node. Indicated in treatment of supraventricular tachycardia, although adenosine has superseded it in urgent situations. Should not be given to patients with wide-complex tachycardia of uncertain origin, because of possible cardiovascular collapse if the rhythm is ventricular	IV dose is 1 mg/min up to a maximum of 10 mg, with continuous EKG monitoring	Avoid in hypotension, secondary and tertiary heart block, significant heart failure and cardiogenic shock, WPW syndrome, porphyria. Commonly causes hypotension on IV administration, particularly in patients with poor LV function. Serious risk of life-threatening bradycardia and asystole in patients recently treated with IV β blockers (risk even exists for oral dose). Therapeutic plasma level 0.1–0.15 µg/mL. Eliminated by hepatic metabolism

Figure 3.17 Continued. ATPase, adenosine triphosphatase; AV, atrioventricular; CNS, central nervous system; EKG, echocardiogram; IV, intravenous; K, potassium; LV, left ventricle; Mg, magnesium; Na, sodium; WPW, Wolff–Parkinson–White (syndrome).

Ventricular arrhythmias
Ventricular tachycardia
CO and blood pressure may be preserved. EKG shows broad-complex tachycardia at 130–250/min with capture and fusion beats. Treatment involves DC cardioversion if hemodynamically compromised (200 J, then 300 J, then 360 J), drugs (eg, amiodarone, lidocaine, others) and overdrive pacing.

Torsade de pointes
This is a variant of VT with alternating polymorphic broad-complex tachycardia. Predisposing factors include a prolonged QT interval, hypokalemia, hypocalcemia, hypomagnesemia, and drugs such as class I antidysrhythmics, tricyclics, phenothiazines.

Treatment involves treating the cause, administration of magnesium sulfate 1–2 g i.v., and treating as for VT.

Ventricular fibrillation
See reference to ACLS guidelines below.

Resuscitation guidelines for adult cardiac arrest
Advanced Cardiac Life Support (ACLS) guidelines were recently revised. The algorithm shown in Figure 3.18 is reproduced from the American Heart Association 2005 guidelines. Further information is available at www.acls.net.

Management of acute heart failure
Heart failure occurs when the heart fails to maintain a CO sufficient for the metabolic needs of the body, or when it can only do so at the expense of abnormally elevated end-diastolic pressures. Heart failure is not a diagnosis as such, but a clinical syndrome; consequently the underlying disease must always be sought and treated.

Chronic heart failure has increased in incidence due to a decline in mortality from acute myocardial infarction, and an increase in the elderly population. It carries a significant mortality risk, with a 5-year survival rate of approximately 30%.

Acute cardiac failure is a medical emergency with a high mortality rate.

Classification of cardiac failure
Left ventricular failure
This is left ventricular impairment, leading to increased end-diastolic volumes and pressures, which causes a raise in pulmonary hydrostatic pressure and

ACLS pulseless arrest algorithm

Pulseless arrest 1
- BLS algorithm: call for help, give CPR
- Give **oxygen** when available
- Attach monitor/defibrillator when available

Check rhythm 2
Shockable rhythm?

Yes → **VF/VT** 3

No → **Asystole/PEA** 9

VF/VT path

Give one shock 4
- Manual biphasic: device specific (typically 120–200 J)
  Note: if unknown, use 200 J
- AMD: device specific
- Monophasic: 360 J
Resume CPR immediately

Give five cycles of CPR

Check rhythm 5
Shockable rhythm?
No

Yes

Continue CPR while defibrillator is charging 6
Give one shock
- Manual biphasic: device specific (same as first shock or higher dose)
  Note: if unknown, use 200 J
- AMD: device specific
- Monophasic: 360 J
Resume CPR immediately after the shock
When i.v/i.o. available, give vasopressor during CPR (before or after the shock)
- **Epinephrine** 1 mg i.v/i.o.
  Repeat every 3–5 min
  or
- May give 1 dose of **vasopressin** 40 U i.v/i.o. to replace first or second dose of **epinephrine**

Give five cycles of CPR

Check rhythm 7
Shockable rhythm?
No

Yes

Continue CPR while defibrillator is charging 8
Give one shock
- Manual biphasic: device specific (same as the first shock or higher dose)
  Note: If unknown, use 200 J
- AMD: device specific
- Monophasic: 360 J
Resume CPR immediately after the shock
Consider **antiarrhythmics**; give during CPR (before or after the shock)
  amiodarone (300 mg i.v/i.o. once, then consider additional 150 mg i.v/i.o. once)
  or **lidocaine** (1 to 1.5 mg/kg first dose, then 0.5–0.75 mg/kg i.v/i.o. maximum 3 doses or 3 mg/kg)
Consider **magnesium** loading dose 1–2 g i.v/i.o. for torsades de pointes
After five cycles of CPR, go to Box 5 above

Asystole/PEA path

Resume CPR immediately for five cycles 10
When i.v/i.o. available, give vasopressor
- **Epinephrine** 1 mg i.v/i.o. **Repeat every 3–5 min**
  or
- May give one dose of **vasopressin** 40 U i.v/i.o. to replace first or second dose of **epinephrine**

Consider **atropine** 1 mg i.v/i.o. for asystole or slow PEA rate. Repeat every 3–5 min (up to three doses)

Give five cycles of CPR

Check rhythm 11
Shockable rhythm?
No

Yes

12
- If asystole, go to Box 10
- If electrical activity, check pulse. If no pulse, go to Box 10
- If pulse present, begin postresuscitation care

Go to 13
Box 4

During CPR

- **Push hard and fast (100/min)**
- **Ensure full chest recoil**
- **Minimize interruptions in chest compressions**
- One cycle of CPR: 30 compressions then 2 breaths; 5 cycles =2 min
- Avoid hyperventilation
- Secure airway and confirm placement

* After an advanced airway is placed, rescuers no longer deliver 'cycles' of CPR. Give continous chest compressions without pauses for breaths. Give 8–10 breaths/min. Check rhythm every 2 min

- Rotate compressors every 2 min with rhythm checks
- Search for and treat possible contributing factors:
  – Hypovolemia
  – Hypoxia
  – Hydrogen ion (acidosis)
  – Hypo-/hyperkalemia
  – Hypoglycemia
  – Hypothermia
  – Toxins
  – Tamponade, cardiac
  – Tension pneumothorax
  – Thrombosis (coronary or pulmonary)
  – Trauma

Figure 3.18 ACLS pulseless arrest algorithm. ACLS, Advanced Cardiac Life Support; AMD, airway management device; BLS, Basic Life Support; CPR, cardiopulmonary resuscitation; PEA, pulseless electrical activity; VF, ventricular fibrillation; VT, ventricular tachycardia. Reproduced with permission from the American Heart Association. *Circulation* 2005; 112:IV1–203.

pulmonary edema. CO may initially be maintained at the expense of increased ventricular stroke work, although ultimately stroke volume falls.

Right ventricular failure

This involves similar processes to the above. Raised filling pressures result in systemic venous hypertension, peripheral edema, hepatomegaly, etc.

Biventricular failure

This occurs either as a result of involvement of both ventricles in the disease process or secondary to left ventricular failure progressively embarrassing right ventricular performance. The latter occurs as a result of:

- raised left atrial pressures and hence pulmonary hypertension, which increases the resistance against which the right ventricle has to work
- left ventricular dilation impinging on right ventricular filling.

High-output heart failure

Certain clinical circumstances (such as arteriovenous malformation, severe anemia, morbid obesity, or thyrotoxicosis) require an increased CO to maintain tissue perfusion. The capacity of the heart to increase CO is limited, and if requirements exceed this capacity then heart failure can develop.

Causes of cardiac failure

The main causes of cardiac failure are the following:

- ventricular outflow obstruction (eg, systemic hypertension, aortic stenosis, pulmonary hypertension, pulmonary stenosis)
- ventricular inflow obstruction (eg, mitral or triscupid valve stenosis, pulmonary embolus, constrictive pericarditis, endocardial fibrosis, and left ventricular hypertrophy)
- ventricular volume overload – increased metabolic demand (eg, hyperthyroidism, sepsis), intracardiac shunting (eg, atrial septal defect), and valvular incompetence (eg, mitral or aortic incompetence)
- impaired ventricular function – diffuse myocardial disease (eg, hypertensive heart disease, myocarditis, cardiomyopathy), focal myocardial disease (eg, ischemic heart disease), and arrhythmias.

Clinical features of acute heart failure

Symptoms:

- dyspnea and orthopnea
- cough, productive of pink frothy sputum

- peripheral edema, abdominal distension
- other features dependent on cause (eg, chest pain in myocardial ischemia, rheumatic fever in cases of valvular heart disease, etc).

Signs:
- tachycardia and third heart sound
- signs of poor CO (eg, cold, clammy skin, sweating)
- elevated jugular venous pressure
- murmurs (eg, mitral regurgitation, aortic incompetence)
- peripheral and sacral edema
- basal inspiratory crackles; in severe cases this may progress to widespread crackles and wheeze (cardiac asthma)
- hepatomegaly (pulsatile in tricuspid regurgitation – transmitted V-wave), ascites
- other signs specific to the underlying cause (eg, endocarditis).

Investigations
Chest X-ray
Pulmonary venous hypertension is marked by vascular engorgement of the upper pulmonary vessels. Interstitial edema is indicated by Kerley B lines (fluid-filled peripheral pulmonary septa) which are never more than 2 cm long and can be seen laterally in the lower lobes. Kerley A lines (edematous central septa) radiate toward the hila in the mid- and upper lobes, they are much thinner than adjacent blood vessels and are 3–4 cm in length. There is a loss of distinction of blood vessels due to fluid collecting around them, edema fluid in lobar fissures, and alveolar edema.

Bat-wing edema is bilateral, involves all lobes, and is maximal near the hila and fades out peripherally.

Cardiomegaly is characterized by dilation of the right or left ventricle which displaces the lower left border of the heart to the left, and therefore does not allow easy distinction between right and left ventricular failure. Cardiomegaly is judged to be present when the maximum transverse diameter of the heart shadow exceeds half of the maximum diameter of the thorax (ie, cardiothoracic ratio >0.5). Globular cardiac dilation is suggestive of pericardial effusion, particularly if the onset is rapid (<2 weeks) and if it is not accompanied by pulmonary edema.

Electrocardiography
EKG can be normal in severe disease, but abnormalities may suggest the cause of heart failure such as:
- left ventricular hypertrophy in hypertensive heart disease

- ischemia/infarction in coronary artery disease
- QRS abnormalities in cardiomyopathy
- arrhythmias.

Echocardiography
The estimated ejection fraction gives an indication of global ventricular function. Regional wall motion abnormalities indicate focal disease (eg, ischemic heart disease). Structural abnormalities (congenital abnormalities, valvular defects, concentric hypertrophy, pericardial effusion) may indicate cause of heart failure.

Other investigations
Alternative investigations to consider include the following:
- a serum chemistry profile – hypo- and hyperkalemia may be associated with arrhythmias, cardiac enzymes, elevated β-type natriuretic peptide levels, hypercholesterolemia in coronary heart disease, abnormal liver function tests in right-sided heart failure
- hematology – anemia may precipitate heart failure, particularly if there is some other underlying heart disease
- thyroid function tests (atrial fibrillation/supraventricular tachycardia)
- blood glucose
- blood cultures (eg, endocarditis).

Management of heart failure
Acute heart failure is a medical emergency, in which diagnosis of the cause and empirical treatment may have to be carried out simultaneously.

Assessment
Peripheral perfusion and pulse can be assessed. It is also important to measure blood pressure, examine jugular venous pressure, and auscultate the lungs and precordium. An intravenous cannula can be inserted and used to take blood for investigations. A 12-lead EKG should be performed; the EKG together with oxygen saturation should be monitored continuously.

General measures
Sit the patient up and administer 35–60% oxygen. Treat ischemic chest pain with nitrates with/without morphine (2.5–5 mg i.v.). In severe cases, a central venous cannula can be inserted to assess filling pressures and allow administration of vasoactive drugs.

Reduction in ventricular afterload

An IV nitrate infusion (eg, 50 mg glyceryl trinitrate in 50 mL saline, 2–10 mL/h) can be administered. A dose of an angiotensin-converting enzyme inhibitor (ACEI) such as captopril, 6.25 mg test dose, increasing to 25 mg every 8–12 h, can also be administered. The initial test dose is necessary due to a risk of severe hypotension (particularly if the patient is also treated with high doses of diuretics). Hyperkalemia may also occur.

Reduction in ventricular preload

Diuretics (eg, furosemide 40–80 mg i.v.) and IV nitrates (administered as above) can be used to reduce ventricular preload.

Inotropic support

Inotropic support is indicated if systolic blood pressure is less than 90 mmHg, particularly if there are signs of organ hypoperfusion (eg, oliguia, confusion, metabolic acidosis). Use dobutamine infusion, starting at 5 mg/kg per min and increasing by 2.5 mg/kg per min every 10 min until systolic blood pressure is more than 95 mmHg, or to a maximum dose of 20 mg/kg per min. It should be given into a central vein. This may cause vasodilatation; an aortic balloon pump counterpulsation may be used to temporarily support a patient awaiting definitive surgical treatment.

Treatment of cause

The list below provides a summary of various treatments that can be used to treat the different causes of acute heart failure:

- thrombolysis in acute myocardial infarction
- anticoagulation in unstable angina
- treatment of arrhythmias as appropriate
- antibiotics in bacterial endocarditis
- drainage of pericardial effusion
- surgical treatment: revascularization, septal defect repair, valve replacement, transplantation.

Unstable angina and acute myocardial infarction

Unstable angina

Unstable angina is defined as angina that:

- occurs with increasing frequency or severity
- occurs at rest or more frequently at night
- is not relieved promptly by nitroglycerine
- is associated with ST depression on the EKG.

Emergency hospital management is based upon the rapid identification and aggressive medical and surgical treatment of patients who are at high risk of death or acute myocardial infarction (AMI). Predictors of high risk include:

- prolonged chest pain at rest (>20 min)
- pulmonary edema
- new/worsening mitral regurgitation
- rest angina with dynamic ST changes of 1 mm or more
- angina with hypotension.

Management of high-risk unstable angina

Admit the patient to the coronary care unit, monitor the EKG continuously, and administer oxygen. Commence nitrate therapy; if no previous nitrates have been given, start with 2–3 sublingual glyceryl trinitrate (GTN) tablets. If the pain persists give 2 mg buccal nitrate, and start intravenous GTN 5–10 mg/h, discontinuing if systolic BP falls below 90 mmHg or by 30% or more.

Further medical management involves administering aspirin 150–300 mg daily (avoid if the patient is allergic, or there is prior intolerance, active bleeding, or severe bleeding risk), or heparin 80 units/kg as intravenous bolus, followed by 18 units/kg per h as an intravenous infusion (avoid if active bleeding, severe bleeding risk, or recent stroke). One can also consider administration of a glycoprotein IIb/IIIa receptor inhibitor. β-Adrenergic blockade can also be administered, atenolol 5 mg i.v. over 5 min, stopping if any complications develop, followed after 10 min by a further 5 mg i.v. provided the heart rate is more than 60 beats/min. An oral dose of 50 mg is given later if the heart rate is more than 50 beats/min, and followed with a further 50 mg after 12 h, then going on to 50–100 mg daily. A dose of morphine 2.5–5 mg i.v. can also be administered, although avoid if the patient is hypotensive or comatose, or the respiratory rate is less than 8 breaths/min.

If chest pain continues despite maximal therapy, urgent angiography should be considered. The majority of patients will have significant stenosis in the distribution of the left coronary artery; these patients will be suitable for either angioplasty or urgent surgical revascularization.

Acute myocardial infarction
Pathogenesis of AMI

Rupture of an atheromatous plaque within the lumen of a coronary artery, and the subsequent formation of fresh thrombus, leads to vascular occlusion and (total) cessation of blood flow to the region of the myocardium supplied by that artery. Hypotension, hypoxemia, and local vasospasm may extend the size of the resulting infarct by compromising the blood supply of surrounding ischemic muscle.

Medical history

There is ischemic pain, typically retrosternal, spreading across the chest, and possibly radiating to the arms, throat, jaw, and back. The pain lasts for more than 20 min and may be atypical (eg, epigastric) which may confuse the diagnosis. A silent (ie, painless) infarction is more common in elderly people and those with diabetes. Many patients give a history of prodromal ischemic symptoms in the preceding days, such as sweating, nausea, dyspnea and orthopnea (particularly in heart failure), and anxiety.

Medical examination

Signs of functional myocardial injury include:
- tachycardia, third or fourth heart sounds, fine inspiratory crackles, elevated jugular venous pressure in heart failure
- hypotension and cold clammy extremities in cardiogenic shock
- dyskinetic apical impulse
- bradycardia in heart block (suggestive of inferior infarct)
- systolic murmur suggestive of mitral regurgitation (papillary muscle rupture or ventricular dilation)
- pericardial friction rub
- fever.

EKG changes in AMI

Less than 10% of patients with enzyme-proven infarcts will have two normal EKGs performed 30 min apart in the hyperacute phase. This establishes electrocardiography as an important initial investigation in the patient with a history suggestive of AMI. The EKG features of AMI are outlined below and are also shown in Figure 3.19.

ST changes

Elevation of the ST segment within the clinical setting of acute ischemic chest pain is believed to represent acute myocardial injury before it evolves into irreversible infarction. Its appearance in the hyperacute phase of AMI gives it a specific role in the indication for thrombolysis or percutaneous revascularization. Reciprocal ST depression is often seen in leads directed away from the injured area, and represents a mirror image of electrical changes rather than additional ischemia. Right ventricular infarction may be identified by ST elevation in the

Correlation between early EKG changes in AMI and coronary artery occlusion		
EKG changes	**Affected region of myocardium**	**Affected artery**
ST depression and tall R-waves in V1–V3	Posterior wall	Right coronary ± left circumflex
ST elevation in II, III, and aVF; reciprocal changes in precordial leads	Inferior wall	Right coronary
ST elevation followed by T-wave inversion in V1–V3	Anteroseptal	Branches of left anterior descending
ST elevation and T-wave inversion in I, aVL, and V4–V6	Anterolateral Massive anterior	Left circumflex Left anterior descending

Figure 3.19 Correlation between early EKG changes in AMI and coronary artery occlusion. AMI, acute myocardial infarction; aVF, arteriovenous fistula; aVL, arteriovenous vein ligation; EKG, electrocardiogram.

V4R lead (ie, the V4 lead placed in the equivalent position on the right side of the sternum). ST changes usually resolve within 2 weeks of injury, although they may persist if a ventricular aneurysm develops. Other causes of ST elevation include pericarditis and coronary vasospasm.

Pathological Q-waves

These are the classic hallmark of an established transmural infarct, with the following characteristics:

- Duration more than 0.04 s.
- Depth more than 4 mm, with a corresponding reduction in size of the ensuing R-wave; a pathological Q-wave is generally more than 25% the height of the R-wave.
- Must appear in leads that do not generally have a Q-wave (eg, have little significance in leads aVR and possibly V1).
- In precordial leads, pathological Q-waves should be associated with QRS complexes which are less than 0.1 s (ie, not left bundle-branch-block [LBBB]).
- Usually present in more than one lead (eg, leads II, III, and aVF in inferior infarction); leads aVL, V5, and V6 in anterolateral infarction, etc.
- Pathological Q-waves may take hours or days to develop following the onset of coronary occlusion. Large Q-waves also occur in hypertrophic obstructive cardiomyopathy and amyloidosis.

T-wave inversion

There are nonspecific signs of ischemia.

Non-Q-wave infarction

This suggests an incomplete (ie, not full thickness) infarct, classically sub-endocardial. The diagnosis is made on the clinical features, an elevation of serum cardiac enzymes, and other EKG changes (eg, T-wave inversion, ST-segment abnormalities), and is important to make since some cases will progress to full-thickness extension without early intervention.

Biochemical changes in AMI

Irreversibly damaged cardiac myocytes release proteins, mainly enzymes, into the circulation, the measurement of which allows confirmation of AMI. The time course of their release varies with the particular marker being assayed.

Myoglobin is a very early marker of cardiac injury, peaking before creatine kinase (CK). Early release may render it a useful guide to thrombolysis. Release from skeletal muscle (eg, following intramuscular injections, trauma) may confuse diagnosis.

Troponins T and I are markers of a hyperacute phase of injury. Troponin T accumulates in renal impairment, possibly limiting its usefulness as an indicator of ongoing myocardial necrosis.

CK peaks at 24 h and disappears after 72 h. Three isoenzymes are recognized:

1. MM (skeletal muscle)
2. MB (myocardium, small intestine, prostate, tongue, uterus)
3. BB (brain).

Measurement of total CK is usually adequate, although the CK-MB fraction may be required in circumstances when other isoenzymes may be released (eg, intramuscular injections, trauma, surgery, defibrillation, muscle disease, exercise, convulsions, cerebral infarction). A CK-MB fraction of 5% or less of total CK indicates significant myocardial injury.

Aspartate transaminase (AST) peaks at 24–36 h, falls within 4–6 days and is less specific than CK. Noncardiac causes of elevated AST include any liver or skeletal muscle injury, pulmonary embolism, and shock.

Lactate dehydrogenase (LDH) peaks at 3–5 days post-infarction, and may take up to 2 weeks to return to baseline. Noncardiac causes of elevated LDH include hemolysis, liver and skeletal muscle injury, various neoplastic disorders (including leukemias), and pulmonary embolism. Five isoenzymes of LDH are recognized, the heart containing principally LDH-1 (the other major source of LDH-1 being erythrocytes). An LDH-1:LDH-2 ratio >1.0 suggests myocardial infarction.

Other investigations in AMI

Echocardiography and coronary angiography can also be carried out. The former allows noninvasive assessment of ventricular performance (including regional motion abnormalities), identification of mural thrombus formation, and characterization of suspected valvular defects. Coronary angiography, is particularly useful in patients in whom emergency percutaneous or surgical revascularization is being considered as a means of limiting infarct size.

Immediate management of AMI

General care involves continuous cardiac monitoring and bed rest for 48 h. Oxygen can be administered via a facemask. Similarly, analgesics such as nitrates, β blockers, or intravenous opioids (eg, morphine 2.5–5 mg) can also be given as required. Administration of a glycoprotein IIb/IIIa receptor inhibitor can be considered. Major trials have demonstrated that intravenous thrombolytic therapy started within 6 h of onset of symptoms significantly reduces mortality in patients with AMI, that there are possible benefits even if this window is extended to 12 h. There are no contraindications to thrombolytic therapy. The indications for thrombolysis in a patient with suspected AMI are chest pain that has lasted for more than 20 min and less than 6–12 h, and EKG changes that show one of the following:

- ST elevation ≥1 mm in two or more of leads I, III, aVL, or aVF
- ST elevation ≥2 mm in two or more of leads V2–V6
- New LBBB
- Signs of true posterior myocardial infarction (ST depression and tall R in V1, ST elevation in V4R).

Contraindications to thrombolytic therapy

Absolute contraindications include:

- major surgery, trauma, or obstetric delivery within the last 2 weeks
- cerebrovascular accident (CVA) or severe head injury within the last 2 months
- previous subarachnoid or intracerebral hemorrhage
- significant gastrointestinal bleeding within the last 2 weeks
- serious active bleeding from any site
- aortic dissection.

Relative contraindications include:

- anticoagulant treatment or bleeding disorder (use rtPA, recombinant tissue-type plasminogen activator, if the international normalized ratio [INR] >3.0)
- proliferative diabetic retinopathy

- prolonged or traumatic cardiopulmonary resuscitation
- pregnancy
- systolic blood pressure >180 mmHg after analgesia
- esophageal varices
- severe liver disease
- active peptic ulceration
- previous CVA with residual disability.

Choice of drug

Streptokinase is the standard agent, and acts by indirectly activating plasminogen. Antibodies raised by previous administration or recent streptococcal infection may limit its effectiveness or cause allergic reactions. Repeat doses should not be given within a 2-year period. It is given as a dose of 1.5 MU in 100 mL 0.9% saline over 1 h. Although there is no current evidence to support anticoagulation following streptokinase therapy, many centers nevertheless administer heparin following thrombolysis.

Alteplase (rt-PA) is an alternate to streptokinase, indications being:
- streptokinase therapy administered within the previous 2 years
- a systolic blood pressure <90 mmHg
- an anterior infarct in patients <70 years old, presenting within 4 h of onset of symptoms.

The dosage regimen is designed to deliver 100 mg alteplase over 90 min as 15 mg by IV injection, followed by 50 mg over 30 min, followed by 35 mg over 60 min. Alteplase should be followed by heparinization in order to help prevent reocclusion, (eg, 2,000 units heparin, followed by 1,000 units/h). Complications of thrombolytic therapy include allergic reactions, hypotension, and bleeding.

Aspirin combined with streptokinase improves the reduction in mortality rate from 25% to 42% by preventing reocclusion of thrombolyzed arteries. A dose of 150–300 mg should be given as soon as possible after the onset of symptoms, and continued daily.

If available, acute percutaneous angioplasty should be considered when thrombolytic therapy is contraindicated, cardiogenic shock, vein graft occlusion, and in specialized centers, as primary therapy for AMI.

β Blockade has a number of potential benefits in patients with AMI. It may reduce the incidence of ventricular arrythmias, afford relief of chest pain, decrease infarct size, lessen the likelihood of cardiac rupture, and reduce mortality overall. It should be given to all patients with suspected AMI (provided that there are no contraindications) as soon as possible. Exclusions to β-adrenergic blockade include:

- asthma and severe chronic obstructive pulmonary disease (COPD)
- pre-existing treatment with β blockers, verapamil, or diltiazem
- heart rate <50 beats/min
- second- or third-degree AV block
- severe heart failure (eg, breathless at rest, fine crackles in the upper zones of the lung).

A suggested regimen for urgent β blockade is atenolol 5 mg i.v. over 5 min, stopping if any complications develop, waiting 10 min, giving a further 5 mg i.v. provided that the heart rate is more than 60 beats/min, stopping if any complications develop, and waiting 10 min. If the heart rate is more than 50 beats/min give atenolol 50 mg orally, and follow with a further 50 mg after 12 h, then give atenolol 50–100 mg/day orally.

Anticoagulation

Alteplase thrombolysis is followed by full anticoagulation with either intravenous heparin or subcutaneous low-molecular-weight preparations (eg, enoxaparin). Patients with large anterior infarcts have a 30% risk of mural thrombus formation, with a subsequent risk of systemic embolization. This group should be given heparin and warfarin on admission, with anticoagulation being discontinued before discharge from hospital if echocardiography fails to reveal a ventricular thrombus. Subcutaneous heparin prophylaxis against thromboembolism, (eg, heparin 5,000 IU every 8–12 h or enoxaparin 40 mg s.c. daily) should be given to patients not formally anticoagulated. As discussed above, aspirin can help prevent reocclusion of thrombolyzed arteries.

Subsequent management and complications of AMI

The in-hospital mortality rate from AMI is now less than 10%, with most deaths occurring within the first few hours, often due to ventricular fibrillation (VF).

Sudden death

Causes of sudden death include:

- asystole
- ventricular tachyarrhythmias
- acute cardiac rupture
- massive pulmonary embolism
- left main stem embolism from mural thrombus.

Suitable monitoring and rapid resuscitation are the keys to successful management of asystole and malignant ventricular arrhythmias. An acute cardiac rupture occurs typically 4–10 days post-infarct, presents with electromechanical dissociation, and is prevented to some degree by early β-adrenergic blockade.

Arrhythmias

VF and pulseless VT should be treated with immediate DC cardioversion. Amiodarone or lidocaine is the treatment of choice for monomorphic VT provided that the patient is hemodynamically stable. Atrial fibrillation can be treated with IV β blockers, amiodarone, or digoxin. Atrial flutter may require DC cardioversion. Patients at risk of late malignant ventricular arrhythmias, occurring 1–3 weeks after infarction, may be identified by early exercise testing or signal averaging of the standard 12-lead EKG (which reveals after-potentials in at-risk individuals).

Bradycardias and heart block

Indications for temporary pacing following AMI include:

- complete AV block
- secondary heart block
- bundle-branch block
- profound sinus bradycardia.

In complete AV block the electrical impulse generated in the atria does not spread to the ventricles. The AV nodal artery is a branch of the right coronary artery (RCA), and complete AV block is therefore more common in inferior infarcts. In the setting of anterior infarcts complete heart block is an indication of massive septal necrosis.

Secondary heart block with a high risk of progression to complete AV block, namely Mobitz type I (Wenckebach) associated with anterior infarction, and any case of Mobitz type II block.

Bundle-branch block is controversial, but indications include the following:

- Trifascicular disease – alternating right bundle-branch block (RBBB) and LBBB, long PR interval + new RBBB + left anterior hemiblock (LAHB), long PR interval + new RBBB + left posterior hemiblock (LPHB), long PR interval + LBBB.
- Nonadjacent bifascicular disease: RBBB + new LPHB. One of the commonest patterns complicating anterior infarction is RBBB + LAHB (presenting as RBBB + left axis deviation) as these two fascicles run in the anterior septum. It only requires pacing if the PR interval becomes prolonged.

Profound sinus bradycardia or sinus arrest if poorly responsive to atropine – this is usually a result of inferior infarction and RCA occlusion.

Heart failure and cardiogenic shock
Heart failure and cardiogenic shock should be managed as indicated elsewhere. Peri-infarct treatment with ACEIs may improve survival, particularly in patients with large infarcts or significant left ventricular dysfunction.

Pericarditis
The accompanying chest pain has a cardiac distribution that is relieved by sitting up or leaning forward, and exacerbated by lying down. A pericardial rub may be heard. The EKG shows 'saddle-shaped' ST elevation with a generalized reduction in voltage if an effusion develops. Treatment is with nonsteroidal anti-inflammatory drugs (NSAIDs).

Systemic embolism
As noted above, patients with large anterior infarcts are at high risk of systemic embolism and should be fully anticoagulated.

Cardiac tamponade
Cardiac tamponade occurs if cardiac rupture is limited to the myocardium and therefore contained within the pericardium. The diagnosis is made by echocardiography and the condition requires urgent surgery.

Mitral regurgitation
Mitral regurgitation is associated with inferior or posterior infarcts. It occurs as a result of papillary muscle dysfunction or rupture, the latter leading to acute and often fulminant pulmonary edema, a loud apical or parasternal pansystolic murmur radiating to the axilla, and cardiogenic shock. Acute valve replacement may be necessary if medical therapy proves ineffective.

Acquired ventricular septal defects
Acquired ventricular septal defects are associated with anterior infarcts. It is difficult to distinguish clinically from acute mitral regurgitation, although right-sided signs predominate with very high venous pressures, and pulmonary edema may be less of a feature. Echocardiography allows the diagnosis to be made, and treatment is urgent surgical repair.

Left ventricular aneurysm
Left ventricular aneurysm may be asymptomatic, although problems include left ventricular failure, refractory angina, recurrent ventricular tachycardia, or systemic embolism. The EKG shows persistent ST elevation, the diagnosis being established by echocardiography or during angiography.

Dressler syndrome
This is a syndrome of recurrent pericarditis, pleural effusions, pyrexia, anemia, and elevated viscosity, which is triggered by the release of myocardial antigenic material following infarction. Treatment is with NSAIDs or steroids in refractory cases.

Cardiogenic shock
Cardiogenic shock is a low-cardiac output state with clinical evidence of inadequate blood flow. It has been defined clinically as a syndrome characterized by hypotension (eg, systolic blood pressure <90 mmHg or 30 mmHg less than normal) or evidence of reduced tissue blood flow (eg, cold clammy skin, urine output <30 mL/h, confusion).

The condition evolves into a vicious circle in which an already seriously impaired ventricle is further embarrassed by reflex neurohumoral sympathetic responses designed to maintain systemic blood pressure and the hypoxia that follows severe pulmonary edema.

Causes
Causes include myocardial infarction, which usually requires loss of at least 40% of muscle mass, myocardial contusions following trauma, tamponade, cardiopulmonary bypass, cardiomyopathy, myocarditis (including rejection of xenograft), and acute valvular dysfunction (including prosthetic valve failure).

Clinical features
These can be grouped accordingly:
- Of the low-output state – cold clammy gray skin, slowed capillary refill time, sweating, confusion, anxiety.
- Of heart failure – elevated jugular venous pressure and other signs of right-sided heart failure, fine inspiratory crackles, tachycardia, and third heart sound consistent with left ventricular failure.
- Of cause – such as chest pain and other features of myocardial infarction, murmurs of acute valvular dysfunction, septal rupture.

Management
General supportive measures

General supportive measures can be carried out, and include continuous monitoring of oxygen saturation and EKG, invasive systemic blood pressure measurement, along with controlled oxygen therapy (with continuous positive airway pressure if pulmonary edema is severe). Central venous cannulation is necessary for the measurement of venous pressures and administration of vasoactive drugs. Intubation and ventilation may be required in the most severe cases. Acid–base status, blood lactate, and hourly urine output should be used as measures of tissue perfusion.

Pulmonary artery catheterization

Insertion of a pulmonary artery catheter gives additional information concerning hemodynamic performance and response to therapy, and can be considered. Most cases of cardiogenic shock are caused by severe left ventricular failure, and will present with pulmonary edema and elevated PAWPs. However, a minority of patients (many of whom present with inferior myocardial infarction) have predominantly right-sided failure, a low PAWP, and an underfilled left ventricle, and consequently require volume loading.

Echocardiography

Echocardiography allows characterization of acute structural alterations such as valvular defects, acquired ventricular septal defects, cardiac rupture, and tamponade.

Hemodynamic management

In cases with preload, if filling pressures are low, increase the plasma volume by administering 200 mL aliquots of colloid solution to maintain PAWP at approximately 18 mmHg. If filling pressures are high, commence infusion of a venodilator such as GTN 0.5–10 mg/h. This may be poorly tolerated in hypotensive patients.

Contractility usually requires inotroptic support, with the aim being to increase arterial blood pressure and thereby improve coronary perfusion pressure. Catecholamines such as dobutamine 2–20 mg/kg per min are generally used. This is probably the agent of choice, although all agents carry the risk of potentiating arrhythmias and worsening myocardial ischemia by increasing cardiac work. Inodilators such as the phosphodiesterase inhibitors are attractive theoretically, although they are arrhythmogenic and less easy to manipulate because of their longer half-lives.

In normotensive patients, with afterload, a reduction in systemic vascular resistance with arteriodilators improves CO and peripheral perfusion. Sodium nitroprusside 10–500 mg/min by IV infusion can be administered. ACEIs are more useful in the recovery phase. Hypotensive patients tolerate arteriodilators poorly unless inotropic support is introduced simultaneously.

Intra-aortic counterpulsation balloon pumping
Intra-aortic counterpulsation balloon pumping improves coronary blood, reduces left ventricular afterload, and increases CO. It is most appropriately used when ventricular performance can be expected to improve (eg, following cardiopulmonary bypass), or as a temporary means of support before cardiac surgery. It may increase the likelihood of successful thrombolysis in patients with cardiogenic shock attributed to AMI.

Cardiac surgery
Surgical revascularization is of little benefit in patients with cardiogenic shock that is a direct result of a massive AMI. It is, however, indicated in patients with acquired ventricular septal defects, acute mitral regurgitation from papillary muscle rupture, and acute cardiac rupture post-MI. It is also indicated in other acute valvular defects (eg, endocarditis-related failure and an obstructing atrial myxoma).

Outcome
The mortality rate of cardiogenic shock overall is around 80%, although this improves to approximately 50% in patients with a surgically correctable lesion. Many survivors are left with significant cardiac pathology such as angina or limiting heart failure.

Chapter 4

The respiratory system

John Kress
University of Chicago, Chicago, IL, USA

The chest X-ray

Figure 4.1 highlights some of the physical signs associated with respiratory disease and Figure 4.2 illustrates the radiological appearance of the lungs in respiratory disease.

Physical signs in respiratory disease					
Condition	**Breath sounds**	**Chest wall movement**	**Mediastinum and trachea**	**Percussion note**	**Tactile vocal fremitus**
Collapse	Increases	Reduced on affected side	Shift to affected side	Dull	Absent
Consolidation	Bronchial breathing, crackles	Reduced on affected side	Central	Dull	Increases
Pleural effusion	Absent, bronchial breathing above fluid level	Reduced on affected side	Shift to opposite side	Dull	Absent

Figure 4.1 Physical signs in respiratory disease.

The following checklist allows a systematic evaluation of a chest X-ray:
1. Name and date.
2. View (posterior-to-anterior views allow more accurate assessment of the size of the heart, but portable anterior-to-posterior films are more common in very sick patients), penetration, rotation (symmetrical position of medial

Radiological appearances of the lungs in respiratory disease

(a) Consolidation of left lung

Mediastinum central (no loss of volume)
Obscured borders of heart/diaphragm

(b) Massive left pleural effusion

Mediastinum and trachea move to right

(c) Collapse of entire left lung

1. Trachea pulled to left
2. Left heart border not seen
3. Left diaphragm obscured
4. Right lung hypertranslucent

(d) Collapse of right upper lobe

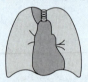

1. Dense wedge in right upper zone
2. Right hilar vessels drawn up and widely spaced
3. Right lower and middle lobes hypertranslucent
4. Trachea and aortic knob pulled to right

(e) Collapse of left lower lobe

1. Dense wedge in heart shadow
2. Left hilar vessels pulled down and widely spaced
3. Left upper lobe hypertranslucent

(f) Right pleural effusion

Note fluid horizontal fissure.
Fluid level not seen if film taken supine; instead the lungfields take on a ground-glass appearance

Figure 4.2 Radiological appearances of the lungs in respiratory disease.

heads of clavicles about the vertebral column), position (usually supine rather than the standard upright film).

3. Review of normal pulmonary volumes: changes in lung volumes are suggested by the following:
    (a) density of lung fields – collapsed areas are more dense, compensatory hyperinflated areas are hypertranslucent
    (b) position of mediastinum
    (c) height and clarity of diaphragm – the diaphragm is often obscured in lower lobe collapse/consolidation
    (d) position of the horizontal fissure and hilar vessels.
4. Regional evaluation of the lung parenchyma:
    (a) upper zone – apex down to lower border of anterior end of second rib
    (b) midzone – between lower borders of anterior ends of second and fourth ribs
    (c) lower zone – lower border of anterior end of fourth rib to diaphragm.
5. Diaphragm and pleura.
6. Heart and mediastinum.
7. Upper abdomen (gas under diaphragm, gastric bubble).
8. Bone.
9. Soft tissues.
10. Special checks:
    (a) apices – pneumothorax, tuberculosis (TB), Pancoast's tumor, upper rib fractures,
    (b) behind heart – metastases, left lower lobe collapse, hiatal hernia.

Hypoxia

Hypoxia is inadequate tissue oxygenation. Its classification can be derived from the factors governing tissue oxygen delivery (DO_2):

$$DO_2 = \text{cardiac output} \times \text{arterial oxygen content}$$

The arterial oxygen content is determined by hemoglobin concentration and arterial oxygen saturation:

$$CaO_2 = 1.39 \times SaO_2 \times [\text{Hb}] + 0.0031 \times PaO_2$$

As can be seen from this formula, the PaO_2 (dissolved oxygen) contributes very little to the arterial oxygen content.

Respiratory failure

The lungs have two major functions: to provide adequate arterial oxygenation for tissue needs and to eliminate CO_2. These two functions are largely independent of each other. Respiratory failure can be classified according to the underlying pathophysiologic derangement. All types of respiratory failure may present with arterial hypoxemia and/or arterial hypercapnia. Mechanisms by which hypoxemia occurs include:

- alveolar hypoventilation (normal A–a gradient is seen only in this setting)
- $\dot{V}/\dot{Q}$ mismatch
- shunt
- decreased mixed venous oxygenation.

Respiratory failure by types

Type I – Acute hypoxemic respiratory failure (AHRF)

This refers to failure of oxygenation due to airspace flooding, which may be caused by alveolar pus (pneumonia), alveolar hemorrhage, or alveolar edema. The last can be further categorized as follows:

- high-pressure edema (eg, congestive heart failure or volume overload)
- low-pressure edema (eg, acute respiratory distress syndrome [ARDS] or acute lung injury [ALI])
- negative pressure pulmonary edema
- re-expansion pulmonary edema
- neurogenic pulmonary edema
- tocolysis-induced pulmonary edema (eg, by administering terbutaline)
- high-altitude pulmonary edema.

Type II – Ventilatory failure

This refers to failure of alveolar ventilation leading to hypercapnia. The arterial $PaCO_2$ is determined by CO_2 production and alveolar ventilation. The difference between alveolar ventilation and minute ventilation ($\dot{V}_E$) is the dead space fraction (V_d/V_t).

$$CO_2 = \frac{(k)(VCO_2)}{[(f)(V_t) \times (1-V_d/V_t)]}$$

where k is a constant equal to 0.863; f is respiratory rate; V_t is tidal volume; V_d/V_t is the dead space fraction.

In this equation, the denominator is the alveolar ventilation. There are three broad mechanisms by which ventilatory failure occurs:

1. Decreased drive to breathe:
    (a) drugs – opiates, benzodiazepines, propofol, barbiturates
    (b) sleep-disordered breathing
    (c) hypothyroidism
    (d) brain-stem lesion (this is a rare cause of decreased drive to breathe).
2. Decreased strength:
    (a) impaired neuromuscular transmission (eg, phrenic nerve injury, spinal cord lesion, neuromuscular blockers, aminoglycosides, Guillain–Barré syndrome, myasthenia gravis, amyotropic lateral sclerosis, poliomyelitis, organophosphate poisoning, botulism)
    (b muscle weakness (eg, fatigue, electrolyte imbalance, malnutrition, hypoxemia, myopathy).
3. Increased load:
    (a) increased airway resistance (eg, bronchospasm, airway edema, secretions, scarring, upper airway obstruction, obstructive sleep apnea)
    (b) decreased lung compliance (eg, auto-PEEP [positive end-expiratory pressure], alveolar edema, infection [lung consolidation], atelectasis)
    (c) decreased chest wall compliance (eg, pleural effusion, pneumothorax, rib fracture, tumor, obesity, ascites, abdominal distension)
    (d) increased minute ventilation load (eg, sepsis, pulmonary embolus, hypovolemia, excessive carbohydrates, shivering, seizures, malignant hyperthermia, thyrotoxicosis).

Type III – Perioperative respiratory failure

A reduction of functional residual capacity below alveolar closing volumes leads to atelectasis:

- supine position
- general anesthesia
- splinting (incisional pain)
- obesity
- ascites
- diminished cough.

Type IV – Shock with hypoperfusion of respiratory muscles

In the normal resting state, 1–5% of the cardiac output is delivered to the respiratory muscles. This can increase up to tenfold in patients with shock and respiratory distress. Mechanical ventilation allows resting of the respiratory muscles.

Noninvasive monitoring

Oxygenation: pulse oximetry

Though arterial blood gas analysis remains the gold standard, noninvasive monitoring of oxygenation with pulse oximetry is used routinely in the critical care setting. This technique takes advantage of differences in the absorptive properties of oxygenated and deoxygenated hemoglobin. At wavelengths of 660 nm, oxyhemoglobin reflects light more effectively than deoxyhemoglobin, whereas the reverse is true in the infrared spectrum (940 nm). A pulse oximeter passes both wavelengths of light through a perfused digit such as a finger, and the relative intensity of light transmission at these two wavelengths is recorded. This allows the derivation of the relative percentage of oxyhemoglobin. Since arterial pulsations produce phasic changes in the intensity of transmitted light, the pulse oximeter is designed to detect only light of alternating intensity. This allows distinction of arterial and venous blood saturations. Though never shown to improve outcomes in the ICU, pulse oximetry is used routinely in virtually every critical care setting as a continuous monitor.

Capnography

Capnography is the analysis of exhaled carbon dioxide (CO_2) concentration. A capnogram measures changes in CO_2 concentration throughout the respiratory cycle. The CO_2 concentration is typically measured with an infrared analyzer that is positioned near the mouth, nose, or the proximal tip of the endotracheal tube. The normal capnogram consists of four distinct portions which are: (A) the ascending limb, (B) the plateau limb, (C) the descending limb, and (D) the baseline (Figure 4.3).

During the baseline portion of the capnogram (D), exhalation of gas from the upper airways (dead space gas) occurs. This gas has no CO_2, so the CO_2

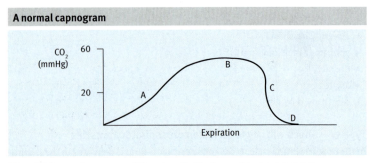

A normal capnogram

Figure 4.3 A normal capnogram. CO_2, carbon dioxide. A normal capnogram showing the ascending limb (A), plateau limb (B), descending limb (C) and the baseline (D).

concentration on the capnogram is zero. Next, as gas from alveoli reaches the infrared analyzer, the CO_2 concentration rises (A). With normal lungs, emptying of alveolar gas is homogeneous, so the rise in CO_2 concentration is rapid and the ascending limb of the capnogram is nearly vertical. In the circumstance of normal physiology, the plateau portion of the capnogram (B) is relatively flat, since alveoli empty in a relatively uniform manner. Heterogeneous empty-ing of lung units results in a more gradual upsloping of the plateau portion of the capnogram. This typically occurs in patients with obstructive airway diseases, such as chronic obstructive pulmonary disease (COPD) or asthma. The end-tidal CO_2, measured at end-expiration (end of portion B in Figure 4.3), is sometimes used as a surrogate for the arterial CO_2. Normally, the difference between end-tidal CO_2 and arterial CO_2 should be less than 5 mmHg – a reflection of the anatomic dead space fraction in normal lungs. Increases in ventilation–perfusion inequalities (which occurs with obstructive airway disease, pulmonary embolism, interstitial lung disease) will result in widening of the gradient between the end-tidal and arterial CO_2 levels.

The descending portion of the capnogram (C) occurs during inspiration; here the CO_2 concentration should rapidly fall to zero, unless rebreathing of CO_2 is taking place. In the ICU, capnography is not used as routinely as pulse oximetry, although it has gained widespread acceptance as a means of confirming suc-cessful endotracheal intubation. Trends in end-tidal CO_2 measurements may be effective indicators of the adequacy of ventilation, even when the end-tidal CO_2 and arterial CO_2 gradients are abnormal because of chronic lung disease.

Oxygen therapy

The oxyhemoglobin dissociation curve has a steep downward portion at a PaO_2 of 60 mmHg (8 kPa) and SaO_2 (percentage of oxygen saturation) of 90% (Figure 4.4). Oxygen therapy should be administered to maintain a SaO_2 of more than 90%.

Methods of oxygen delivery
Variable-performance devices

These systems deliver modest flows of oxygen (1–15 L/min) via a simple semi-rigid facemask or nasal cannulae. Since the delivered flow is consider-ably less than the peak inspiratory flow rate (25–30 L/min at rest, rising to more than 60 L/min in dyspneic states), room air is entrained and the oxygen is diluted to a variable and unpredictable extent. The precise oxygen concentration is therefore unknown. Such systems are classified according to their capacity to store oxygen during the expiratory pause and thereby enrich the oxygen/air mixture of the subsequent inspiration.

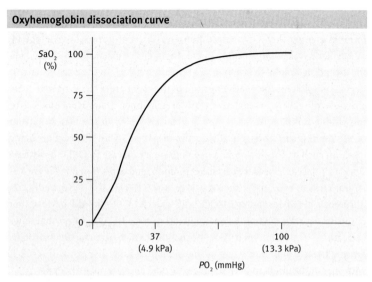

Figure 4.4 Oxyhemoglobin dissociation curve. PO_2, partial pressure of oxygen; SaO_2, percentage oxygen saturation.

Nasal cannulae are well tolerated, and allow the patient to continue to eat and drink. They do not increase dead space, and therefore there is no possibility of rebreathing expired CO_2. At oxygen flows of 1–2 L/min there is little or no storage of oxygen in the nasopharynx during the expiratory pause, and therefore cannulae behave as a no-capacity variable-performance device. At flows of 2–4 L/min, significant storage of oxygen may occur, and so a higher concentration of oxygen can be achieved. High flow rates can damage the nasal mucosa.

Semi-rigid plastic facemasks are examples of variable-performance devices with a small capacity. A minimum flow rate of 4 L/min is required to flush expired gas from the mask chamber and thereby prevent rebreathing of expired CO_2. At higher flow rates oxygen accumulates within the mask and enriches the oxygen content of the subsequent breath.

Soft plastic masks with a reservoir bag have a much larger capacity to store oxygen during the expiratory pause and can therefore support higher inspired oxygen concentrations when used with oxygen flow rates of 10–15 L/min. If lower flow rates are used considerable rebreathing of expired gas accumulating within the large reservoir bag may occur. They are very useful in resuscitation to maximize the FiO_2 (inspired oxygen fraction) in spontaneously ventilating patients.

The approximate oxygen concentrations achieved with some devices are shown in Figure 4.5, which shows that the oxygen concentration with 'open'

Oxygen concentrations achieved with variable-performance devices			
Oxygen delivery system	Intended oxygen concentration (%)	Tracheal oxygen concentration (%)	
		Quiet breathing	Hyperventilating
Facemask			
10 L/min	60	53.4	41.0
15 L/min	100	68.1	50.2
Nasal cannula			
3 L/min	–	22.4	22.7
10 L/min		46.2	30.5
15 L/min		60.9	36.2
Venturi mask	28	24.2	21.4
4 L/min	40	36.4	29.4
8 L/min			

Figure 4.5 Oxygen concentrations achieved with variable-performance devices.

breathing systems can vary widely. Oxygen concentration can be known precisely only with 'closed' breathing systems (eg, endotracheal tube or tight-fitting facemask connected to a mechanical ventilator).

Mechanical ventilation

Clinical applications

Clinical applications can be summarized as follows:

- cardiopulmonary resuscitation
- respiratory failure
- postoperative ventilation following major surgery, to permit correction of homeostatic disturbances before the patient awakens (eg, hypothermia, electrolyte imbalance, profound anemia)
- severe sepsis, when the patient is unable to meet the increased work of breathing demanded by high CO_2 production and metabolic acidosis
- control of $PaCO_2$ as part of the management of severe intracranial hypertension (eg, head injuries).
- support ventilation in patients requiring endotracheal intubation to protect/maintain the airway
- reduction of cardiac work in cardiogenic shock.

Indications

Objective criteria for consideration of mechanical ventilation include:

- respiratory rate >35 mmHg
- oxygenation: PaO_2 <60 mmHg (8 kPa) on 60% oxygen
- ventilation: $PaCO_2$ >60 mmHg (8 kPa) accompanied by arterial pH <7.3.

Clinical assessment is, however, more important than objective criteria, using the following features:

- Respiratory system: breathlessness, tachypnea, open-mouth breathing, irregular respiration, heaving respiration, abnormal inspiration:expiration ratio, inspiratory lag, ineffective cough, active expiration, holding bedframe, lifting arms, sweating, flaring alae nasi, pursed mouth, cyanosis, difficulty in talking, moaning, grunting, requesting ventilator, head off pillow, active accessory muscles, noisy or wheezing respiration.
- Central nervous system: drowsiness, restlessness, anxiety, apathy, exhaustion, disorientation, weak smile, picking bedclothes.
- Cardiovascular system: cooling of extremities (nose, ears, hands, feet), rising pulse, dysrhythmia, falling blood pressure, rising venous pressure, falling urinary output.

If in doubt transfer to the ICU, as a sudden deterioration requiring ventilation can be dealt with more efficiently and safely here than on a ward.

Complications of ventilatory support

Hemodynamic instability occurs particularly when starting positive pressure ventilation. It is caused by the depressant effects of sedative drugs, inhibition of the thoracic pump that promotes venous return, and blunting of endogenous catecholamine release. High inflation pressures and PEEP exaggerate these effects, which are worse in patients with hypovolemia.

Acid–base disturbances such as respiratory acidosis or alkalosis are possible if minute volume is incorrectly set. Long-term hyperventilation reduces the buffering capacity of the cerebrospinal fluid (CSF) so that during weaning any increase in $PaCO_2$ leads to an unexpectedly large fall in the pH of the CSF, which may result in dyspnea.

In respiratory muscle atrophy, full mechanical ventilation may lead to isuse atrophy of the respiratory muscles; subsequent weaning will thus be more difficult.

Pulmonary barotrauma, exposure of the lungs to plateau airway pressures greater than 30 cmH_2O, *may* increase the risk of ventilator-induced lung injury, although the evidence supporting this supposition is controversial. Damage appears to be a result of the shear forces generated when collapsed lung units are repeatedly reinflated during inspiration as well as alveolar overdistension. PEEP may help prevent such injury by keeping units open throughout the respiratory cycle. Prolonged overdistension of lung units with large tidal volumes may lead to lung injury indistinguishable from ARDS. Strong evidence supports the use of low tidal volume ventilation in the context of ALI to avoid alveolar overdistension.

Complications of endotracheal intubation, and laryngeal and pharyngeal injury, may occur when endotracheal tubes have been in place for longer than 3 weeks. The presence of an endotracheal tube prevents satisfactory mouth hygiene, which in turn may lead to the microaspiration of (infected) pharyngeal fluids, and so cause nosocomial pneumonia. Sedation is regularly required to facilitate endotracheal intubation (particularly via the oral route). Nasotracheal intubation carries a high risk of sinusitis. For complications of sedation see Chapter 2.

Modes of ventilatory support

Volume-controlled modes

The clinician sets the tidal volume and respiratory rate. The ventilator delivers whatever pressure is needed to achieve the set tidal volume.

Controlled mandatory ventilation

Controlled mandatory ventilation (CMV) is similar to ventilation during surgery. Respiratory rate and tidal volume/minute ventilation are determined by the clinician. CMV is used when little or no spontaneous respiratory effort by the patient is desired (eg, in critical hypoxia).

Assist-control ventilation

The clinician sets the tidal volume and respiratory rate. The ventilator delivers at least the number of tidal volumes each minute. Spontaneous breaths in between preset breaths are assisted with the full preset tidal volume. It is often used when the goal is to minimize the work of breathing.

Synchronized intermittent mandatory ventilation (SIMV)

The clinician sets the tidal volume and respiratory rate and the ventilator delivers exactly that number of tidal volumes each minute. These mandatory breaths re synchronized with the patient's spontaneous efforts (ie, if a mandatory breath is due to be delivered when the patient is spontaneously inhaling, the mandatory breath is delayed until exhalation is finished, thereby preventing breath 'stacking'). All spontaneous breaths between mandatory breaths are unassisted.

Pressure-controlled modes

The clinician sets the maximal inspiratory pressure and the ventilator delivers whatever tidal volume is generated by that pressure. A preset pressure is applied to the airways at a preset rate and preset inspiration:expiration ratio. Pressure-controlled ventilation is used to limit airway pressures when low lung compliance might otherwise lead to the risk of barotrauma. Delivered tidal volume varies with changes in compliance and resistance, and minute ventilation is therefore variable.

Pressure support

This is the spontaneous breathing mode with no preset breaths. Positive pressure is applied to the airways in response to inspiratory effort. The tidal volume delivered depends upon the compliance of the respiratory system (lungs and chest wall) and airway resistance, and therefore varies. It is generally started at 20–30 cmH$_2$O and reduced as the patient's respiratory mechanics improve. It is sometimes combined with SIMV to assist spontaneous breaths in excess of the preset rate, although evidence of beneficial outcome using this strategy is lacking. In proportionally assisted ventilation the applied inspiratory pressure is proportional to the inspiratory effort of the patient. Volume-assured pressure support is an alternative in which the inspiratory pressure is automatically varied by the ventilator to achieve a preset tidal volume.

Positive end-expiratory pressure and continuous positive airway pressure

These techniques employ baseline elevations of the airway pressure during mechanical (PEEP) and spontaneous (continuous positive airway pressure [CPAP]) ventilation. It is used to improve oxygenation by redistributing alveolar edema to the pulmonary interstitium and to improve respiratory mechanics by restoring reduced lung volumes to normal.

Other modes of mechanical ventilation

Inverse-ratio ventilation

The respiratory cycle (the time devoted to the delivery and exhalation of one mechanical breath) is divided into inspiratory and expiratory times. Normal inspiration:expiration ratios are 1:2 to 1:3. The relative prolongation of the inspiratory time (so-called inverse-ratio ventilation) is often used to improve gas exchange in patients with poor oxygenation. A ratio of 2:1 to 3:1 is commonly used. This method can be applied to either pressure- or volume-controlled ventilation.

Noninvasive ventilation

Various devices are now available to apply positive pressure to the airways via a tightly fitting mask (either nasal or full face). These are used to apply CPAP with or without additional support during inspiration, avoiding the need for endotracheal intubation.

Liberation from mechanical ventilation

Patients who have been ventilated for brief periods of time (eg, overnight ventilation following major surgery) may be liberated from mechanical ventilation rapidly in a manner similar to practice in the operating room (namely termination of sedation, then a brief period of time breathing on a T-piece or a rebreathing circuit, followed by extubation). This is in marked contrast to patients who have been critically ill for long periods of time (days), in whom the process of withdrawing ventilatory support is often protracted. Day-to-day changes in the patient's condition during this period of respiratory convalescence often necessitate the temporary reintroduction of more substantial mechanical ventilatory support.

Quoted measures of respiratory function associated with successful liberation include the following:

1. Measures of oxygenation: PaO_2/FiO_2 (>150–200).
2. Measures of capacity and load on the respiratory system (though these parameters have been traditionally quoted, none is particularly sensitive or specific for predicting successful liberation):
   (a) V_d/V_t (<0.6)
   (b) tidal volume >5 mL/kg
   (c) vital capacity >10 mL/kg
   (d) respiratory system compliance (>25 mL/cmH$_2$O)
   (e) respiratory system resistance (<20 cmH$_2$O/L/s)
   (f) maximum inspiratory force >−20 to 30 cmH$_2$O
   (g) respiratory rate <35 breaths/min
   (h) minute ventilation <10–15 L/min
   (i) maximum voluntary ventilation (>twice minute ventilation).
3. Integrative index: frequency-tidal volume ratio (<105 breaths/min per L).

Clinical assessment is important, and mirrors the features of respiratory distress indicating ventilatory impairment at the inception of respiratory failure. Factors associated with liberation difficulties include:

- persistence of the primary pathology
- untreated cardiovascular or renal failure
- malnutrition
- sepsis or pyrexia (increased metabolic demands)
- fluid overload
- residual sedation
- delirium/coma
- electrolyte imbalance (particularly Ca^{2+}, Mg^{2+}, K^+, PO_4^{3-})
- anemia

- pain
- abdominal distension.

Most patients are able to breathe spontaneously as soon as the cause(s) of respiratory failure is treated. Studies have shown that daily spontaneous breathing trials (breathing on CPAP or T-piece) can effectively identify patients ready for liberation from mechanical ventilation. The spontaneous breathing trial is the best predictor of successful liberation from mechanical ventilation. The patient passes a screening process if:

1. PaO_2/FiO_2 >200
2. PEEP <5
3. Cough and airway reflexes intact
4. Frequency to tidal volume ratio <105
5. No vasopressor agents or sedatives, spontaneous breathing trial with CPAP 5 cmH$_2$O or T-piece for 30–60 min is indicated.

The patient fails if:

1. Respiratory rate (RR) >35 for >5 min
2. SpO$_2$ <90%
3. Heart rate >140 or 20% change from baseline in either direction
4. Systolic BP <90 or >180 mmHg
5. Clinical evidence of increased anxiety, diapheresis.

If none of these events occurs the patient should be evaluated for extubation. If there is a good cough, no evidence of excessive swelling around the endotracheal tube (eg, passing a cuff deflation test), and the patient is neurologically intact sufficient to protect the airway, extubation should be performed. Tracheostomies aid weaning, particularly in patients who have been ill for some time. One study demonstrated that early tracheostomy reduced many complications of critical illness. The advantages of tracheostomy include:

- Reduced sedation requirements – most patients require little or no sedation in order to tolerate a tracheostomy, in contrast to endotracheal tubes which are very stimulating.
- Improved nutrition – largely a result of reduced sedation.
- Improved oropharyngeal toilet – may reduce incidence of nosocomial pneumonia.
- Reduced airway resistance.
- Easier access to lower respiratory tract secretions.
- Flexibility with changes in respiratory support.

Management of respiratory failure

Type I – Acute hypoxemic respiratory failure (AHRF)

Patients exhibit shunt physiology. Hypoxemia typically requires high FiO_2 and PEEP. Attempts should be made to keep FiO_2 lower than 60% to avoid oxygen toxicity to the lungs:

1. Alveolar edema:
   (a) high-pressure edema:
      · congestive heart failure – diuretics, inotropes, angiotensin-converting enzyme inhibitor (ACEIs)
      · volume overload – diuretics, renal replacement therapy in renal failure.
   (b) low pressure edema (eg, ARDS or acute lung injury [ALI]):
      for a more detailed discussion see the section on ALI/ARDS.
2. Alveolar pus (pneumonia): focal alveolar pus may lead to inflammation that overwhelms hypoxic pulmonary vasoconstriction. PEEP may overdistend normal alveoli without affecting consolidated lung, thereby worsening gas exchange. See section on pneumonia for a more detailed discussion.
3. Alveolar hemorrhage: often occurs in patients with coagulation disturbances, especially thrombocytopenia. Bone marrow transplant recipients are also at risk. May be seen in various collagen vascular diseases and vasculitides. Treatment is centered around supportive care of AHRF, as outlined below, as well as treatment of coagulation disturbance. Treatment of specific vasculitides (eg, Wegener's granulomatosis) with corticosteroids and cytotoxic agents (eg, cyclophosphamide) may be curative.

Discussion of common causes of respiratory failure

Acute lung injury and acute respiratory distress syndrome

Definition and etiology

ARDS is a syndrome causing acute respiratory failure characterized by severe hypoxemia, poorly compliant ('stiff') lungs, and diffuse patchy infiltration on the chest X-ray in patients in whom cardiogenic pulmonary edema has been excluded. Rather than being an isolated condition, it is recognized as the pulmonary manifestation of systemic inflammation. ARDS is now recognized as the extreme end of a spectrum of ALI, and is defined in terms of the severity of the gas exchange defect (Figure 4.6). Also required for diagnosis is exposure to a recognized cause of ALI, which can be either direct or indirect (Figure 4.7).

Acute lung injury versus ARDS

	Acute lung injury	ARDS
Chest X-ray	Bilateral infiltrates	Bilateral infiltrates
Onset	Acute	Acute
PaO_2 (mmHg)/FiO_2	<300	<200
Pulmonary artery wedge pressure (mmHg)	<18	<18

Figure 4.6 Acute lung injury versus ARDS. ARDS, acute respiratory distress syndrome. FiO_2, inspired oxygen fraction; PaO_2, partial pressure of oxygen.

Causes of acute lung injury

Direct	Indirect
Smoke/toxin inhalation	Sepsis
Aspiration of gastric contents	Systemic inflammation and MODS
Near drowning	Anaphylaxis
Thoracic trauma	Cardiopulmonary bypass
Diffuse pulmonary infection (eg, *Pneumocystis jiroveci*)	Neurogenic pulmonary edema
	Non-thoracic trauma
	Pancreatitis
	Fat embolism
	Massive transfusion
	Air embolism

Figure 4.7 Causes of acute lung injury. MODS, multiple organ dysfunction syndrome.

Clinical features

The early stages of ALI are characterized by pulmonary edema. This is a result of an inflammatory process centered around the pulmonary microcirculation, which leads to an increase in the permeability of the alveolar–capillary barrier. The alveolar flooding that follows leads to atelectasis, poor lung compliance, gas exchange abnormalities, and pulmonary hypertension. This inflammatory stage is followed by a period of proliferative repair in which destruction of normal lung architecture ends in fibrotic destruction, microvascular obliteration, and increases in dead space. The mortality rate of ARDS ranges from 30% to 40%, and has improved significantly in recent years with the advent of new ventilator strategies.

Management

Ventilator management strategies showing survival benefit were established from the recent ARDSnet (ARDS network) trial as follows:

- mode – volume control (assist control)

FiO_2 and PEEP titration values from the ARDSnet trial

FiO_2	0.3	0.4	0.4	0.5	0.5	0.6	0.7
PEEP	5	5	8	8	10	10	10
FiO_2	0.7	0.7	0.8	0.9	0.9	0.9	1.0
PEEP	12	14	14	14	16	16	20–24

Figure 4.8 FiO_2 and PEEP titration values from the ARDSnet trial. ARDSnet, acute respiratory distress syndrome network; FiO_2, inspired oxygen fraction; PEEP, positive end-expiratory pressure.

- tidal volume – 6 mL/kg *ideal* (not actual) body weight
- FiO_2 and PEEP – see Figure 4.8
- plateau airway pressure – <30 cmH_2O. If plateau airway pressure >30 cmH_2O despite 6 mL/kg tidal volume, further decrease to lower tidal volume (down to 4 mL/kg ideal body weight).

PEEP helps to redistribute alveolar edema into the pulmonary interstitium, thereby improving gas exchange.

Fluid restriction/diuresis limits increases in pulmonary capillary hydrostatic pressure and therefore lung water. A fluid conservative approach (eg, CVP <4 mmHg) has been shown to shorten duration of mechanical ventilation without worsening renal function.

Prone ventilation may improve $\dot{V}/\dot{Q}$ relationships by directing blood flow away from previously dependent atelectatic areas. With prone positioning, approximately 70% of patients improve oxygenation, although no survival benefit has been demonstrated.

The case for steroids is unproven, although some authorities advocate the use of pulsed methylprednisolone to prevent the progression to the destructive fibrotic phase of the disease.

Community-acquired pneumonia

Pneumonia can be defined as an acute lower respiratory tract illness, which is associated with fever, symptoms and signs in the chest, and abnormalities on the chest X-ray. In patients admitted to the hospital, it carries an overall mortality of about 10%. Mortality is strongly correlated with age, chronic comorbidities, severely abnormal vital signs upon presentation, and laboratory abnormalities (eg, pH, blood urea nitrogen, Na^+, glucose, hemoglobin, and PaO_2).

Clinical features
- fever
- cough and purulent sputum

- pleuritic chest pain
- dyspnea
- tachypnea
- signs of collapse, consolidation, airway obstruction.

Classification

Anatomic:

- lobar pneumonia
- bronchopneumonia
- diffuse.

Pattern of illness:

Typical: a sudden onset and a lobar distribution (eg, *Streptococcus pneumoniae*, *Klebsiella* spp., *Hemophilus* spp.).

Atypical: gradual onset, with a diffuse patchy distribution (eg, *Mycoplasma* spp., *Legionella* spp., *Chlamydia* spp., *Coxiella* spp., viral).

Epidemiologic:

- community acquired
- hospital acquired
- immunodeficiency related.

Microbiology:

Understanding of the likely pathogens in given circumstances is an important guide to empiric antibiotic therapy.

Assessment of severity

Identification of a severe form of pneumonia is important, because it not only indicates an increased risk of death, but also dictates more aggressive antibiotic therapy. Features of severe pneumonia are the following:

- Clinical features: respiratory rate 30/min, diastolic blood pressure 60 mmHg, age 60 years, underlying disease states, confusion, multilobar involvement.
- Laboratory features: serum urea 42 mg/dL, serum albumin 3.5 g/dL, PaO_2 60 mmHg (8 kPa), white blood cell count 4,000 × 10^9/L or 20,000 × 10^9/L, bacteremia.

Investigations

Several investigations can be carried, these include:

- A chest X-ray: consolidation and collapse, cavitation, effusion, cardiomegaly and heart failure, and pre-existing respiratory disease

- Arterial blood gas analysis: can be used in cases of chronic respiratory disease (eg, compensated respiratory acidosis), hypoxemia, and acid–base status
- A complete blood count: anemia as an indicator of chronic disease, hemolysis, white cell count (high or low) as an index of severity of infection. Platelet count may be low in severe sepsis as part of a consumptive coagulopathy
- Urea and electrolytes: renal function is often deranged in severe sepsis, and as a specific feature of *Legionella* infection
- Liver function tests (including clotting studies): assessment of severity of sepsis, or indicator of severe underlying disease.

Microbiological tests of the sputum, blood, urine and pleural fluid can also be carried out.

In the sputum, paired Gram-positive cocci suggest pneumococci while clusters of Gram-positive cocci suggest staphylococci. The incidence of community acquired meticillin-resistant *S. aureus* is increasing. Special stains are available for mycobacteria (eg, Ziehl–Neelsen), *Legionella* spp., influenza and respiratory syncytial virus (RSV) (eg, immunofluorescence), *Pneumocystis* spp. (eg, silver stain, immunofluorescence). Prior antibiotic therapy may prevent successful culture of causative organisms. Difficult diagnostic problems (eg, severe pneumonia of unknown cause, the presence of normal upper respiratory tract organisms in tracheal aspirates from intubated patients) may justify invasive procedures to obtain samples from the lower respiratory tract, eg, bronchoscopy with bronchoalveolar lavage, and protected specimen brush.

Positive blood cultures are usually diagnostic. Serology is used for influenza A and B, RSV, adenovirus, *Coxiella burnetii, Chlamydia psittaci, Mycoplasma pneumoniae,* and *Legionella pneumophila*. A fourfold rise in titers is diagnostic, although it often develops too late to be of clinical importance. A raised *Mycoplasma*-specific IgM titer is usually seen on admission in patients with *M. pneumoniae.*

Urinary tests to carry out are a *Legionella* antigen test. The pleural fluid can also be tested; microscopy and culture of bacterial organisms, and a pH <7.2 are suggestive of empyema.

Indications for transfer to the ICU

The following are all indications for transferring a patient to the ICU:

- two of the following: respiratory rate 30/min, diastolic BP 60 mmHg, urea 42 mg/dL
- PaO_2 <60 mmHg (8 kPa) with inspired oxygen at 60%
- $PaCO_2$ >48 mmHg (6.4 kPa) (suggesting respiratory fatigue), unless chronic CO_2 retainer (will have compensated respiratory acidosis)

- exhaustion
- respiratory arrest
- evidence of shock/organ hypoperfusion (eg, hypotension persisting despite fluid challenge, metabolic acidosis, oliguria, confusion)

Management and monitoring of severe pneumonia

Monitoring should ideally take place in an ICU environment, and include:

- continuous EKG and pulse oximetry monitoring
- noninvasive blood pressure measurements
- arterial cannulation to allow regular arterial blood gas analysis, and continuous blood pressure recording
- respiratory rate
- urine output and fluid balance (fluid overload may lead to pulmonary edema, further compromising gas exchange).

Oxygen therapy should be sufficient to maintain arterial oxygen saturation >90–93%. Chest physiotherapy in patients without coexisting lung disease is of uncertain value, but may benefit patients with a depressed conscious level when sputum retention may lead to lobar collapse, etc. For antibiotic therapy see below.

Antibiotic therapy

Antibiotic therapy should commence as soon as the diagnosis has been made, usually before the identity of the infective agent is known (Figure 4.9). Such empiric therapy depends upon the severity of the illness, likely pathogens, coexisting medical conditions such as COPD or heart disease, and the known sensitivities of likely respiratory pathogens in the local community (eg, incidence of ampicillin-resistant *Hemophilus influenzae*). Specifically, it should:

- always cover *S. pneumoniae*
- include a macrolide antibiotic if *Legionella* or *Mycoplasma* is suspected
- include an anti-staphylococcal agent during an influenza epidemic
- be modified when microbiological information becomes available
- be continued for at least 5 days, and possibly longer if recovery is slow (patients with *Legionella* or *Staphylococcus* spp. may require treatment for 2 weeks or more).

Failure of an infective episode to resolve raises the possibility of:

- incorrect diagnosis: pulmonary embolus, heart failure, connective tissue disorders, etc
- resistant organism

- pulmonary tuberculosis
- empyema and pulmonary abscess
- underlying malignancy, immunodeficiency
- anatomic abnormality – post-obstructive pneumonia.

Health-care-associated pneumonia

A new category defined as pneumonia developing in the following types of patients:

- Hospitalized in an acute care hospital for >2 days within 90 days of the infection
- Nursing home or long-term acute care resident
- Recipient of IV antibiotics, chemotherapy, or wound care within the past 30 days of the current infection
- Regular visits to hospital or hemodialysis clinic
- Health-care-associated pneumonia is included in the spectrum of hospital-acquired and ventilator-associated pneumonia. Therapy directed at multidrug-resistant pathogens is necessary.

Hospital-acquired (nosocomial) pneumonia

This is defined as pneumonia developing more than 2 days after admission to hospital. It is particularly common in the ICU and postoperative patients, and carries a mortality rate of up to 50%. Likely infecting organisms include the following:

- Gram-negative bacilli: *Pseudomonas aeruginosa*, *Enterobacter* spp., *Klebsiella pneumoniae*, *Escherichia coli*, *Serratia marcescens*, *Proteus mirabilis*, *Acinetobacter* spp., *Hemophilus influenzae*
- Gram-positive cocci: *Staphylococcus aureus*, *Streptococcus* spp.
- Fungi: *Aspergillus* spp.

Many of these organisms colonize the upper respiratory and gastrointestinal tracts before infection, and aspiration of such infective material into the lower respiratory tract has been proposed as an important mechanism in the evolution of nosocomial pneumonia.

Diagnosis

Diagnosis often proves difficult, particularly in ventilated patients, because features are nonspecific and may be confused with other conditions (eg, heart failure, aspiration pneumonitis, ALI). Contamination of tracheal aspirates with organisms that have colonized the upper respiratory tract and major airways is a particular problem. Nevertheless, the current (ideal) recommendation is to

Forms of pneumonia

Organism	Notes	Antibiotic treatment[†]
Chlamydia psittaci	2–3% of cases. Recent contact with (sick) bird	1. Azithromycin 500 mg i.v. q day 2. Ciprofloxacin 400 mg i.v. b.i.d.
Coxiella burnetii	Causes Q fever. Pneumonitis following infection acquired from ticks resident in animal hides. Rarely associated with endocarditits or hepatitis	As for *Mycoplasma pneumoniae*
Gram-negative bacilli (*Klebsiella, Pseudomonas, Escherichia coli*)	Rare in community-acquired pneumonias. More common in patients with chronic illness, and important causes of hospital-acquired pneumonia. Treatment should be guided by sensitivities and local hospital antibiotic policies wherever possible	1. Second- or third-generation cephalosporin, eg, cefotaxime 2 g i.v. t.i.d. 2. Ciprofloxacin 200–400 mg i.v. b.i.d. or ceftazidime 1–2 g i.v. t.i.d. if *Pseudomonas* spp. likely 3. Aminoglycoside 4. Anti-pseudomonal penicillin, eg, piperacillin, plus an aminoglycoside
Hemophilus influenzae	5% of all cases, more frequently as an infective exacerbation of pre-existing lung disease. Resistance to ampicillin increasing	1. Ceftriaxone 1–2 g i.v. q day 2. Cefotaxime 1–2 g i.v. t.i.d.
Legionella spp.	Typically in middle-aged men, and more common in immuno-suppressed patients. Responsible organism often found in ventilation and air-conditioning systems. More common in summer/autumn; suspect particularly if recent hotel stays, contacts, etc. Renal and cardiovascular system complications are common and the mortality is relatively high	1. Azithromycin 500 mg i.v. q day + rifampicin 600 mg i.v. b.i.d.
Mycoplasma pneumoniae	5–20% of all cases. Often prodromal flu-like illness, commonly in children/ young adults. Diffuse opacification on chest X-ray. Nonpulmonary complications uncommon. Recovery often protracted	1. Doxycycline 100 mg i.v. q 12 h 2. Azithromycin 500 mg i.v. q day

Figure 4.9 Forms of pneumonia. [†]1, first-line antibiotic; 2, alternative; 3, third-line antibiotic; 4, fourth-line antibiotic.

Forms of pneumonia (*continued*)

Pneumocystis spp.	Rare, although important cause of respiratory failure in immuno-compromised individuals. High mortality	1. Trimethoprim/ sulfamethoxazole 5 mg TMP/ kg i.v. q 6 h (total of 20 mg TMP/day) 2. Pentamidine 4 mg/kg i.v. daily for at least 14 days. Reduce dose in renal impairment. Side effects (such as severe hypotension) are reduced by inhalational administration
Staphylococcus aureus	Up to 5% of all cases. Important cause of pneumonia following influenza, measles; also common following aspiration (head injuries etc). Sputum shows clusters of Gram-positive cocci. Cavitation and abscess formation can occur	1. Vancomycin 1 g i.v. q 12 h (until MRSA ruled out) 2. Nafcillin 1 g i.v. q 4–6 h if not MRSA
Streptococcus pneumoniae	Up to 60% of all community-acquired pneumonias. Paired Gram-positive cocci. Usually lobar distribution; pneumococcal meningitis rare	1. Ceftriaxone 1–2 g i.v. q day 2. Benzylpenicillin 1–2 g i.v. q day 3. Azithromycin 500 mg i.v. q day if allergic to penicillin
Viral Influenza virus Other viruses		1. Oseltamivir 75 mg p.o. b.i.d. x 5 days for those symptomatic <2 days (influenza A and B) 2. Rimantadine 100 mg p.o. b.i.d. (100 mg p.o. q day for age >65)

Figure 4.9 Forms of pneumonia (*continued*). MRSA, meticillin-resistant *Staphylococcus aureus*; TMP, 2,2,4-trimethylpentane.

obtain a lower respiratory culture (bronchoscopically or nonbronchoscopically) prior to beginning antibiotic therapy. However, antibiotic therapy must not be delayed while cultures are obtained. The diagnosis of ventilator-associated pneumonia is described in Figure 4.10.

Management

If empiric therapy is required then all samples for microbiology (blood, sputum, and possibly pleural fluid) should be obtained before it starts. Treatment should be guided by local antibiotic policies, previous antibiotic treatment, and known local variations in prevalence and antibiotic sensitivities, as well as the implications of specific clinical situations (Figure 4.11).

Diagnosis of ventilator-associated pneumonia	
Definite diagnosis	**Probable diagnosis**
1. Radiological evidence of pulmonary abscess plus positive needle aspirate culture 2. Histological and quantitative infection following open lung biopsy	1. Positive blood culture within 48 h of culturing of identical organism from respiratory tract 2. Positive quantitative culture from microbiologic evidence of lower respiratory tract using a technique that minimizes contamination with upper respiratory tract flora, such as bronchoalveolar lavage, protected brush specimens 3. Culture of the same organism from sputum and pleural fluid 4. Histologic evidence of pneumonia without positive quantitative microbiology

Figure 4.10 Diagnosis of ventilator-associated pneumonia.

Pulmonary tuberculosis

This should always be considered in patients failing to respond to conventional antibiotic therapy. Risk factors include:

- patients from a developing country
- poverty, malnutrition
- alcoholism
- HIV infection and other causes of immunosuppression
- close contact with smear-positive patients.

Clinical features include lassitude, anorexia, weight loss, productive cough, and night sweats. There may be coexisting chronic bronchitis. Mortality in patients requiring admission to the ICU is high.

Diagnosis

1. Sputum, bronchial lavage, or gastric lavage specimens for microscopy for acid-fast bacilli (Ziehl–Neelsen stain)
2. Transbronchial and pleural biopsy
3. Chest X-ray:
   (a) normal X-ray excludes TB (except in HIV)
   (b) commonly presents with patchy/nodular shadowing in upper zones, cavitation, calcification, lymphadenopathy, pleural effusions, or diffuse infiltration (miliary TB).

Management

During the initial phase (1–2 months) the following are administered together:
   (a) isoniazid 300 mg daily

Antibiotic therapy for nosocomial pneumonia

Situation	Likely organisms	Therapeutic options
Mild–moderate illness, no specific risk factors	Core organisms: *S. aureus,* *Klebsiella* spp. *Enterobacter* spp. *E. coli,* *Proteus* spp. *Serratia* spp. *H. influenzae*	Core antibiotics: 1. Cefazolin plus gentamicin 2. Second-generation cephalosporin (eg, cefuroxime) 3. Non-pseudomonal third-generation cephalosporin (eg, cefotaxime) or ciprofloxacin 4. β-Lactam/β-lactamase inhibitor combination (eg, co-amoxiclav)
Mild–moderate illness: Aspiration Thoracoabdominal surgery	Core organisms, anaerobes	1. Core antibiotics plus metronidazole 2. β-lactam/β-lactamase inhibitor combination
Coma, head injury	Core organisms, especially *S. aureus,* *Hemophilus* spp.	Core antibiotics plus antistaphylococcal agent (eg, nafcillin). Meticillin-resistant strains require vancomycin
High-dose corticosteroids	Core organisms plus *Legionella* spp.	Core antibiotics plus azithromycin
Multiple risk factors (including prolonged hospital stay, previous broad-spectrum antibiotics, ICU admission) and severe pneumonia	Core organisms plus *P. aeruginosa, Acinetobacter* spp.	1. Anti-pseudomonal penicillin (eg, piperacillin) plus aminoglycoside 2. Anti-pseudomonal cephalosporin (eg, ceftazidime) plus aminoglycoside or quinolone (eg, ciprofloxacin) 3. Imipenem/cilastin

Figure 4.11 Antibiotic therapy for nosocomial pneumonia. ICU, intensive care unit.

(b) rifampin 600 mg daily (450 mg if <50 kg)

(c) pyrazinamide 2 g daily (1.5 g if <50 kg) plus ethambutol (if drug resistance likely) 25 mg/kg daily.

Throughout the continuation phase (3–12 months), the following administered:

(a) isoniazid 300 mg daily

(b) rifampin 600 mg daily (450 mg if <50 kg) plus ethambutol (if drug resistance likely) 15 mg/kg daily.

Ethambutol causes a dose-dependent loss of visual acuity that is exacerbated by renal impairment.

Diagnosis of ventilator-associated pneumonia

Diagnosis requires new airspace opacity on chest X-ray, purulent tracheal aspirate, plus fever, and/or increased white blood cell count with left shift often seen.

Pneumonia in the immunocompromised host

Patients with HIV or hematological malignancies, and bone marrow transplant recipients are at a particular risk of pneumonia.

Bacterial infections tend to develop more rapidly than fungal pneumonias (Figure 4.12). A suggested empiric regimen for febrile neutropenic patients is:

1. Third-generation antipseudomonal cephalosporin (eg, ceftazidime) plus IV aminoglycoside; evaluate after 72 h:
   (a) if fever subsides and patient improves, continue for 1–2 weeks
   (b) if patient remains febrile but is clinically improving, continue for 7 days and add amphotericin B
   (c) if patient fails to respond, add vancomycin and amphotericin B on day 7.
2. If chest X-ray changes are diffuse, add co-trimoxazole plus azithromycin.
3. Consider vancomycin earlier if MRSA or coagulase-negative staphylococci (line sepsis) are likely.

Pneumocystis jiroveci (formerly Pneumocystis carinii) pneumonia

This has an insidious onset, with fatigue, weight loss, dry cough, fever, and respiratory failure. The chest X-ray shows diffuse bilateral perihilar

Chest X-ray appearances and likely organisms	
Focal infiltrates	**Diffuse infiltrates**
Gram-negative rods	Cytomegalovirus
S. aureus	Herpes virus
Mycobacterium tuberculosis	Advanced fungal infections
Aspergillus and other fungal infections	Pneumocystis spp.
Legionella	
Pneumocystis spp. (rarely)	

Figure 4.12 Chest X-ray appearances and likely organisms.

shadowing, although initially it may be normal. Mortality is high but improving. The diagnosis depends on a high index of suspicion. Bronchoalveolar lavage provides a cytological diagnosis in most cases. It may be possible to avoid bronchoscopy by inducing bronchorrhea and sputum production with nebulized hypertonic 3% saline. Treatment is started as soon as the diagnosis is suspected:

- Trimethoprim/sulfamethoxazole: 20 mg/100 mg per kg daily for 3 weeks (reducing dose by 25% if white cell count falls) **or** pentamidine 4 mg/kg i.v. for 3 weeks
- Prednisone: 40 mg b.i.d. for 5 days, then 20 mg b.i.d. for 5 days, then 20 mg daily thereafter
- Second-line drugs: clindamycin 600 mg i.v. four times daily + primaquine 15–30 mg orally daily, or trimetrexate 45 mg/m^2 i.v. + leucovorin 20 mg/m^2 i.v. four times a day.

Aspiration syndromes

Etiology

Impaired conscious level:

- head injury
- coma
- anesthesia
- drugs (including alcohol)
- seizures
- cerebrovascular accident.

Impaired gag/cough reflexes:

- bulbar palsy (Guillain–Barré syndrome, motor neuron disease, multiple sclerosis, etc.)
- pharyngeal trauma
- recent extubation.

Passive regurgitation:

- pregnancy
- hiatus hernia
- anesthesia associated with esophageal/gastric outlet/intestinal obstruction
- emergency anesthesia in patients with a full stomach
- esophageal surgery
- nasogastric tubes (large)
- achalasia, scleroderma.

Pathophysiology

A number of aspiration syndromes are recognized.

1. Aspiration of solid material blocking laryngeal inlet: this medical emergency is treated with maneuvers such as the Heimlich maneuver, the finger sweep, laryngoscopy and intubation, or surgical airway (emergency cricothyroidotomy, etc).
2. Aspiration of solid material blocking a major bronchus (dental fragments, peanuts, coins, food, etc) causes atelectasis and bronchiectasis distal to obstruction. It requires bronchoscopic removal. Secondary infections should be treated with drainage and antibiotic therapy.
3. Aspiration of gastric acid (in a previously well, nonhospitalized patient) may result in a chemical pneumonitis, particularly if the pH of the gastric contents is less than 2.5. It carries a high mortality. Clinical features include dyspnea, bronchospasm, pulmonary edema, hypoxia, and shock. Management is as follows:

    - The patient should be placed head down on the right side, and the oropharynx cleared of any remaining material.
    - Administer oxygen.
    - Intubate if the level of consciousness is impaired, or if respiratory failure develops.
    - Monitor cardiorespiratory function, including continuous pulse oximetry, and EKG.
    - Pass nasogastric tube to empty stomach.
    - Treat bronchospasm with nebulized β_2 agonists.
    - Cardiovascular collapse may result from the loss of blood plasma from the pulmonary microcirculation and the accompanying SIRS – establish arterial and central venous access to guide intravascular fluid resuscitation. Pulmonary artery catheterization may be necessary in severe cases to guide fluid therapy and inotropic support as required.
    - Perform baseline chest X-ray: therapeutic bronchoscopy is indicated if there is any clinical or radiological evidence of lobar/lung collapse or the presence of a foreign body; therapeutic lavage is not useful.
    - Avoid prophylactic antibiotics if there is no reason to believe that the stomach contents included pathogenic bacteria (patient previously well, not hospitalized, not on antacids, etc). Secondary infection may, however, develop. If it is necessary to treat before bacteriological confirmation, use third-generation cephalosporin (eg, cefotaxime) + nafcillin + metronidazole. A carbipenem (eg, imipenem) is a suitable alternative.

4. Aspiration of infected gastric/intestinal fluid can occur. As a result of low pH, gastric fluid is usually sterile. However, increases in pH resulting from antacid or H_2-receptor antagonist therapy lead to overgrowth of stomach contents with intestinal microorganisms, particularly in patients who are hospitalized and unwell. Aspiration of such material, although not causing such severe pneumonitis, delivers a considerable inoculum of pathogens into the lungs. Patients present with pneumonia/respiratory failure. Alternately the changes may be diffuse. Features of pneumonitis (aspiration, pulmonary edema, shock) may be absent, and the development of respiratory failure may be insidious. Respiratory failure should be dealt with appropriately. Broad-spectrum antibiotics should be started, and provide cover against anaerobes, S. aureus, and Gram-negative species, including Pseudomonas spp. Although intubated patients are relatively protected against macroscopic aspiration, continuous microaspiration of infected gastric fluid past the cuff of an endotracheal tube probably accounts for many of the nosocomial pneumonias seen in this group.

5. Aspiration of hydrocarbons following the accidental ingestion of organic fluids such as petrol or turpentine may cause a severe ALI. Treatment is supportive.

Fat embolism

Fat embolism is an uncommon condition in which the intravascular deposition of fat globules leads to respiratory and neurological failure.

Cutaneous manifestations (petechial hemorrhage, known as livedo reticularis) complete the triad. It is traditionally considered to result from the release of fat emboli from bone marrow or adipose tissue, although some believe that it may be caused by changes in the solubility of circulating lipids. Causes of fat embolism include:

- orthopedic trauma
- pancreatitis
- liposuction
- parenteral nutrition
- bone marrow transplantation.

The syndrome is dominated by respiratory failure. Plugging of the pulmonary microcirculation leads to gas exchange abnormalities, pulmonary hypertension, and cor pulmonale. A severe inflammatory response to the fat emboli leads to pulmonary vasculitis and pneumonitis with resulting AHRF (type I respiratory failure). Platelet sequestration and the subsequent release of vasoactive compounds such as 5-hydroxytryptamine add to the inflammatory process.

Clinical features
- Systemic: pyrexia, tachycardia, jaundice, retinal hemorrhage.
- Pulmonary: dyspnea, tachypnea, cyanosis, diffuse infiltration on chest X-ray.
- Neurological: headache, confusion, coma, convulsions.
- Cutaneous: petechial rash (livedo reticularis), particularly in chest, axillae, conjunctiva.
- Laboratory: anemia, thrombocytopenia, coagulation abnormalities.

Diagnosis
Diagnosis of fat embolism is clinical. Appearance of fat globules in the urine is neither sensitive nor specific.

Management
- Early fixation of fractures.
- Cardiorespiratory support as necessary (mechanical ventilation with PEEP is required in severe cases).
- A number of pharmacologic therapies such as corticosteroids, ethanol infusions, albumin, and aprotonin have been suggested, although there is no firm evidence to support their use.

Prognosis
The condition is self-limiting and has a mortality rate of around 10%.

Acute severe asthma
Acute asthma is an inflammatory disease of the airways in which an initial phase of constriction of the bronchial smooth muscle is followed by airway mucosal edema and bronchial plugging. Acute severe asthma usually develops in patients with poorly controlled asthma and persistent airway obstruction. Response to β_2 agonists is often poor, but the condition improves with steroids. Hyperacute fulminant asthma develops more rapidly, often in individuals with little or no chronic airway limitation. It may be life threatening within minutes but responds quickly to aggressive bronchodilator therapy.

Features of acute severe asthma
- unable to finish a sentence in one breath
- respiratory rate >25/min
- heart rate >110/min
- peak expiratory flow rate (PEFR) <50% predicted normal or recorded best.

Features of life-threatening asthma (status asthmaticus)

- PEFR <33% predicted normal or recorded best
- silent chest, cyanosis, feeble respiratory effort
- exhaustion, confusion, coma
- bradycardia, hypotension
- normal or rising $PaCO_2$, acidosis, falling PaO_2.

Immediate management of status asthmaticus

- Oxygen – highest flow and concentration available.
- Nebulized β_2 agonist every 15 min, in a volume of 2–4 mL – albuterol 2.5 mg in 3 mL saline, may require continuous albuterol nebulization.
- Methylprednisolone 125 mg i.v. every 6 h – peak response at 6–12 h, but should be given immediately.
- Measure arterial blood gases; obtain chest X-ray.
- Continuous clinical observation is mandatory: this should be supplemented by continuous pulse oximetry and intermittent measurement of peak flows and arterial blood gases. Check plasma electrolytes – hypokalemia is likely.
- Avoid sedation or physiotherapy. Antibiotics are indicated only if there is a clear evidence of purulent bronchitis or pneumonia.

Intensive care

Patients with life-threatening asthma should be transferred to the ICU with continuous SaO_2 and EKG monitoring. Arterial access facilitates arterial blood gas analysis. Indications for mechanical ventilation are as follows:

- exhaustion
- depressed conscious level
- falling respiratory rate not associated with clinical improvement
- rising $PaCO_2$.

  Noninvasive ventilatory support such as mask or nasal CPAP ventilation may delay or avoid the need for intubation and invasive mechanical ventilation in some patients.

Mechanical ventilation

The phenomenon of gas trapping or pulmonary hyperinflation is the principal difficulty encountered during status asthmaticus. Obstruction of expiratory airflow means that, unless the time for expiration is increased, expiration may be incomplete when the next breath is delivered. Both the lung and intra-alveolar pressure at the end of expiration will rise as a result.

Pulmonary hyperinflation in asthma

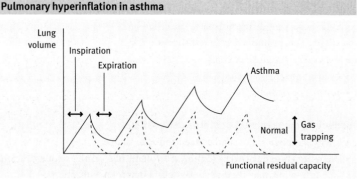

Figure 4.13 Pulmonary hyperinflation in asthma.

This phenomenon is known as auto-PEEP or intrinsic PEEP. Obstruction to inspiratory flow means that higher peak airway pressures will be superimposed on these elevated end-expiratory pressures (Figure 4.13). Ventilatory strategies include the following:

1. Deep sedation.
2. Small tidal volumes, limiting plateau inflation pressures to <30 cmH_2O (6–8 mL/kg).
3. Long inspiratory and expiratory times, leading to low respiratory rate.
4. Points (2) and (3) above imply low minute volumes and therefore rising $PaCO_2$. Such permissive hypercapnia is an acceptable alternative to more aggressive ventilation, which would expose the lungs to higher inflation pressures.
5. An awareness of the continued risk of gas trapping and pneumothorax. Sudden rises in airway pressures may be caused by pneumothorax.

In refractory cases consider the following:

- Epinephrine may be considered in addition to conventional β_2-agonist therapy. Administer either as intravenous infusion or by nebulizer. Continuous EKG monitoring is mandatory (high risk of tachyarrhythmias).
- Heliox (gas mixture of helium 80%:oxygen 20%) is a low density gas that decreases transpulmonary pressure required to deliver equivalent volume compared with oxygen:nitrogen mixtures. It may also change gas flow from turbulent to laminar thus decreasing work of breathing.
- Magnesium sulfate 5–10 mmol (2.5–5 mL 50% solution) over 20 min; hypotension may develop.
- Montelukast 7–14 mg i.v. has been shown to be beneficial in a randomized trial.

Acute deteriorations in chronic obstructive pulmonary disease

Pathophysiology

In COPD, destruction of the elastic tissues of the airways and hypertrophy of the bronchial mucosa result in reduced elastic recoil and increased airway resistance, respectively. The net result is increased resistance to expiratory airflow, which causes pulmonary hyperinflation and reduced mechanical efficiency of the respiratory muscles. The work of breathing therefore increases.

Parenchymal disease leads to $\dot{V}/\dot{Q}$ mismatching, with increased dead space. Hypoxic pulmonary vasoconstriction worsens pulmonary hypertension, which can precipitate right-sided heart failure. Increases in dead space demand corresponding increases in minute volume if adequate elimination of CO_2 is to be maintained. The work of breathing is therefore further increased.

Chronic hypoxia leads to secondary polycythemia. Failure of respiratory muscles to support the increased minute ventilatory requirements leads to CO_2 retention.

Two extreme clinicopathologic extremes are identified: chronic bronchitis and emphysema. Although they usually coexist, a description of the clinical features of each is useful (Figure 4.14).

Causes of acute respiratory failure in COPD (acute-on-chronic respiratory failure):

- infection (bronchitis, pneumonia)
- sputum retention (post-operative, concurrent illness)
- bronchospasm
- pneumothorax and bulla formation
- heart failure
- dysrhythmias
- pulmonary embolism
- end-stage COPD.

Management

For oxygen therapy, administer oxygen to maintain $SaO_2 > 90\%$. Many physicians are taught to avoid giving high oxygen concentrations to patients with COPD. This recommendation is based upon the notion that these patients rely on a hypoxic drive to breathe and that administering supplemental oxygen decreases the drive to breathe. Several studies have refuted this hypothesis. Patients with COPD given supplemental oxygen may have an increase in $PaCO_2$, but this is a consequence of worsening $\dot{V}/\dot{Q}$ mismatch, not hypoventilation.

Clinical features of chronic bronchitis and emphysema	
Chronic bronchitis	**Emphysema**
Chronic productive cough	Little cough/sputum
Wheeze	Continuous and progressive dyspnea
Fluctuating dyspnea	Progressive increases in dyspnea
Profound $\dot{V}/\dot{Q}$ abnormalities $\rightarrow$ hypoxia and hypercapnia	Less profound $\dot{V}/\dot{Q}$ disturbances
Frequent (infective) exacerbations and remissions	
End stage is 'blue bloater' – pulmonary hypertension and cor pulmonale, polycythemia, CO_2 retention. May be complicated by obstructive sleep apnea	End stage is 'pink puffer'

Figure 4.14 Clinical features of chronic bronchitis and emphysema. CO_2, carbon dioxide; $\dot{Q}$, perfusion; $\dot{V}$, ventilation.

Bronchodilator and steroid therapy involves administering the following:
- nebulized ipratropium bromide 0.5 mg in 2 mL saline every 2–6 h
- nebulized albuterol 2.5 mg in 3 mL saline every 2–4 h
- methylprednisolone 125 mg i.v. every 6 h.

Antibiotics can be used to treat severe community- or hospital-acquired pneumonia as appropriate.

Effective clearance of secretions is crucial, and is best achieved by regular and frequent physiotherapy (every 2–4 h). Pharyngeal suction may be useful when conscious level is impaired.

Coexisting heart failure should always be suspected, particularly in patients failing to respond to conventional therapy. Treat with diuretics; afterload reduction with ACEIs. Consider spironolactone if renal insufficiency is not an issue. Avoid β blockers.

Look for and correct electrolyte disturbances, particularly hypokalemia, hypomagnesemia, and hypophosphatemia; ensure adequate nutrition.

Early administration of noninvasive mask ventilation with CPAP usually starts at 3–5 cmH_2O. Alternately, use bilevel positive airway pressure with inspiratory driving pressures starting at 3–5 cmH_2O and end-expiratory pressures starting at 3–5 cmH_2O. These may be titrated up to patient response and comfort. A tight, properly fitting mask is crucial for success with noninvasive positive pressure ventilation.

Indications for endotracheal intubation include: fatigue, despite noninvasive ventilation; acute respiratory acidosis, despite noninvasive ventilation; coma, inability to protect airway; sputum retention; and cardiorespiratory arrest. Avoid rapid reductions in $PaCO_2$ when introducing ventilatory support, and be prepared to treat the cardiovascular instability that is often seen at this time. Weaning from ventilation can be difficult and may require early tracheostomy.

Pulmonary embolism

Pulmonary embolism (PE) occurs in 15–20 patients per 1,000 of the general hospital population, of which 2–5 cases are fatal. At least 50% of patients who die from PE have had some indication of thromboembolism within the preceding 7 days. Failure to diagnose PE has adverse consequences, since 30% of patients with untreated PE die compared with 8% of treated PE.

Etiology

Pulmonary emboli usually result from the formation of asymptomatic deep vein thromboses (DVTs) in deep veins of the lower limbs, pelvis, and abdomen. Upper extremity DVTs are usually associated with indwelling catheters and may account for up to 15% of DVTs. Calf DVTs rarely embolize, although propagation to more proximal site is common, so they should be treated. Factors promoting the formation of thrombi are described by Virchow's triad of venous stasis, abnormal vessel walls, and increased coagulability (Figure 4.15).

Virchow's triad		
Venous stasis	**Abnormal vessels**	**Increased coagulability**
1. Immobility	Trauma	Polycythemia
Old age	Phlebitis	Thrombocytopathy
Obesity	Previous DVT	Sickle cell disease
Perioperative		Hyperviscosity syndrome
Severe illness		Protein C, S deficiencies
Stroke		Smoking
Spinal injury		Malignancy
Guillain–Barré syndrome		Pregnancy
Trauma		Oral contraceptive pill/estrogen therapy
2. Reduced flow		
Cardiogenic shock		
Myocardial infarction		
Pregnancy		
Pelvic tumors		
Perioperative venous occlusion		

Figure 4.15 Virchow's triad. DVT, deep vein thrombosis.

Pathophysiology

PE typically causes partial occlusion of the pulmonary vasculature. Because of recruitment and distensibility, at least 50% occlusion is necessary to cause pulmonary hypertension. Hypoxia, vasoactive amine release, and neural reflexes add to the pulmonary arterioconstriction. A massive PE results in acute right heart failure: increased afterload due to pulmonary artery occlusion/vasoconstriction, hypoxia, and acidosis.

Alterations in lung mechanics such as bronchoconstriction and atelectasis, occur possibly a result of loss of surfactant.

Gas exchange defects: increase in alveolar dead space means that minute ventilation must increase to maintain effective clearance of CO_2 and oxygenation is often disturbed; however, 37% of patients with PE have a PaO_2 >70 mmHg; increases in shunt fraction result from the continued flow of blood through atelectatic areas. $\dot{V}/\dot{Q}$ abnormalities develop due to the redistribution of pulmonary blood flow through a smaller lung volume (increasing perfusion in relation to ventilation).

Pulmonary edema is occasionally seen, possibly due to the loss of surfactant and increase in pulmonary artery pressures. This is not common.

Clinical features

Clinical evidence of a DVT is uncommon. Clinical features of the embolus depend upon its size:

- Small embolus – may have no features; recurrent small emboli cause progressive dyspnea, cor pulmonale, and fever.
- Medium-sized embolus – there is dyspnea, subsequent pulmonary infarction causes pleuritic chest pain, hemoptysis, and pleural effusions.
- Large embolus – this is defined as an embolus involving the blood supply to two or more lobes. Clinical features include: acute cor pulmonale (tachycardia, elevated jugular venous pressure, loud pulmonary second sound and gallop rhythm, right ventricular heave), hypoxemia, and shock. Dyspnea, tachypnea, and central chest pain are also present as well as occasionally bronchospasm and crackles.

Investigations

Blood tests to carry out include a *d*-dimer test as *d*-dimer levels are usually elevated; levels <500 mg/L virtually exclude diagnosis. In the ICU population, this is not sensitive since *d*-dimer levels are usually elevated for other reasons. Bilirubin, white cell count, and lactate dehydrogenase levels may also be elevated.

A chest X-ray is often normal; however, focal oligemia (Westermark's sign), atelectasis, a large proximal pulmonary artery, and a dilated right ventricle due to large emboli may also be present. Smaller emboli cause wedge-shaped infarcts and pleural effusions.

EKG may be normal. Tachycardia and tachydysrhythmias may also be seen. ST depression and T-wave inversion in the anterior chest leads (V1–V4) indicate right ventricle (RV) strain. A classic picture of a deep S-wave in I, with a Q-wave and T-wave inversion in III (SIQIIITIII) is rare.

An echocardiogram will show RV strain and dilation. Occasionally, emboli may be seen in the pulmonary artery or right ventricle. The size of the left ventricle is also reduced. Echocardiography is a useful bedside investigation for RV syndromes.

Spiral CT of the thorax is a noninvasive investigation commonly used in critically ill patients. It was originally reported to have a sensitivitiy and specificity greater than 95%, but more recent trials suggest this is closer to 70%.

A $\dot{V}/\dot{Q}$ scan is a traditional noninvasive investigation, in which radioisotopes are used to define areas of pulmonary hypoperfusion and establish whether or not they are associated with corresponding areas of hypoventilation. The result is expressed as a probability. A normal perfusion scan excludes PE. However, any underlying cardiorespiratory disease will significantly weaken the power of the examination.

Pulmonary angiography remains the 'gold standard' diagnostic test for PE. The mortality rate in large series is less than 2%.

As many as 30% of patients with PE will have evidence of a DVT. Techniques to identify a DVT include: Doppler ultrasound, impedance plethysmography, venography, and magnetic resonance imaging.

Decision-making guidelines

The decision to treat a suspected PE can be difficult to make. A suggested decision pathway is shown below.

Occasionally, in patients in whom the clinical suspicion of a large PE is very high, anticoagulation with heparin before confirmation is justified. When a moderate-to-large embolus is suspected, a bedside echocardiogram should be obtained to look for right heart dysfunction. If a moderate or large embolus is suspected, a spiral CT (if available) will demonstrate proximal (but not small peripheral) pulmonary emboli. If these diagnostic options are not available or, if a small PE is suspected, one may perform a $\dot{V}/\dot{Q}$ scan. If this is negative then search for a DVT (using Doppler ultrasound, venogram, etc); if a proximal DVT is present, then anticoagulate.

Treatment

- Small PE: oxygen, fluids, anticoagulation (see below). For recurrent small PEs treatment is as above or a caval filter can be implanted.
- Massive PE: oxygen, mechanical ventilation for respiratory failure, circulatory support, (eg, maintain high CVP, inotropes – dobutamine, norepinephrine may help, pulmonary artery catheter may help to manage fluid and inotropic therapy), and anticoagulation/thrombolysis (Figure 4.16).

Anticoagulation

Heparin prevents further fresh thrombus formation and inhibits propagation of the established embolus. It may also attenuate the release of vasoactive compounds within the pulmonary circulation, and thereby limit pulmonary hypertension. The dose is a loading dose of 80 units/kg unfractionated IV heparin followed by continuous infusion of 18 units/kg per h. Keep activated partial thromboplastin time (APTT) 1.5–2.5 × normal. Subcutaneous low-molecular-weight heparin may be just as effective as IV unfractionated heparins (eg, enoxaparin 1 mg/kg every 12 h). However, this has not been studied extensively in the critically ill patient. Alternatives to heparin include heparinoids such as lepirudin (renally cleared and contraindicated in renal failure) and argatroban (hepatically cleared).

Warfarin is introduced once the patient is stable. Heparin is continued until adequate warfarinization, as measured by the international normalized ratio (INR), has been achieved. Suggested target INRs are as follows:

- DVT prophylaxis in high-risk surgery: 2–2.5
- prophylaxis in hip surgery: 2–2.5
- treatment of DVT/PE: 2–3
- treatment of recurrent DVT/PE: 3.

Initially INR should be measures daily and then on alternate days. Warfarin is continued for 1.5–2 months in patients with proven DVT and 3–6 months following PE.

Systemic thrombolysis		
Drug	**Dose**	**Comments**
Streptokinase	Loading: 250,000 IU over 30 min Maintenance: 100,000 IU/h for 24 h	Antibodies from previous exposure or streptococcal infection may reduce effectiveness and increase the risk of allergic reactions and anaphylaxis
rtPA	100 mg over 2–3 h	Expensive but no antibody formation

Figure 4.16 Systemic thrombolysis. rtPA, recombinant tissue-type plasminogen activator.

Reversal of warfarin

Acute reversal of warfarin therapy is best achieved with fresh frozen plasma. Reversal with large doses of vitamin K (<10 mg) interferes with subsequent attempts to re-warfarinize for 2–3 weeks; small doses (0.5–1 mg) may be effective and yet avoid these problems. Warfarin must be stopped at least 3–4 days prior to elective surgery.

Thrombolytic therapy

Thrombolytic therapy is indicated for massive PE with associated shock. Its role in massive PE, with echocardiographic evidence of right heart failure or massive PE with severe pulmonary hypertension, has demonstrated improved secondary outcomes compared with heparin, though no survival benefit has been noted.

Allergic reactions and hemorrhage are the principal complications of thrombolytics, and restrict their use considerably. Contraindications are shown in Figure 4.17. Regimens for systemic thrombolysis are shown below. Unnecessary venepuncture should be avoided and intramuscular injections are contrain-

Contraindications for thrombolytics
Absolute
Recent puncture in a noncompressible site
Active or recent internal bleeding
Hemorrhagic diathesis
Recent CNS surgery or active intracranial lesion
Uncontrolled hypertension (BP >180/110 mmHg)
Known hypersensitivity for streptokinase, use within 6 months
Diabetic hemorrhagic retinopathy
Acute pericarditis
Recent obstetric delivery
History of stroke
Relative
Trauma (including CPR) or major surgery within 10 days
Pregnancy
High likelihood of left heart thrombus
Infective endocarditis
Advanced age
Liver disease
Alcoholism
Renal insufficiency

Figure 4.17 Contraindications for thrombolytics. BP, blood pressure; CNS, central nervous system; CPR, cardiopulmonary resuscitation.

dicated. Heparin should be recommenced once the thrombolytic therapy has been completed. In the event of serious hemorrhage:

- stop infusion
- give fresh frozen plasma
- in the case of streptokinase therapy, give aprotinin 500,000 IU or ε-aminocaproic acid 5–8 g.

Other measures

Inferior vena caval filters can be used, although complications such as migration, caval wall erosion, and inferior vena cava obstruction limit their use. Indications include:

- recurrent PE despite anticoagulation
- inability to tolerate anticoagulation therapy
- large thrombus in iliofemoral system
- following pulmonary embolectomy.

Acute pulmonary embolectomy should be considered in patients with persistent hemodynamic compromise in whom thrombolytic therapy has failed or is contraindicated. This procedure carries a high risk of mortality.

Acid–base balance and blood gas analysis

The pH scale encompasses an enormous range of hydrogen ion concentration (H^+) and is not particularly well suited to the description of biological acidity:

$$DO_2 = \text{cardiac output} \times \text{arterial oxygen content}$$

The range of H^+ compatible with life is 20–160 nmol/L; a pH change of 0.3 unit is equivalent to a doubling or halving of H^+:

- pH 6.8 = 160 nmol/L H^+
- pH 7.1 = 80 nmol/L H^+
- pH 7.4 = 40 nmol/L H^+
- pH 7.7 = 20 nmol/L H^+.

Biologic buffering systems

A buffer is a substance that has the capacity to minimize the pH change that the addition of an acid or base would otherwise produce. The effectiveness of a particular buffering system is determined by its concentration, the pK_a – of the buffer (the pH at which the buffer is 50% ionized – the closer this is to the biologic pH the more effective it is), and whether other physiological mechanisms can restore the concentration of the buffering activities (Figure 4.18).

Biochemical features of acid–base disturbances

	Respiratory		Metabolic	
	Acidosis	**Alkalosis**	**Acidosis**	**Alkalosis**
Primary disturbance	Increased $PaCO_2$	Decreased $PaCO_2$	Increased H^+ or decreased HCO_3^-	Increased HCO_3^-
Acute response	$CO_2 + H_2O \rightarrow$ [HCO_3^-] rises by 1 mmol/L for each 10 mmHg rise in $PaCO_2$ [H^+] rises by 8 nmol/L for each 10 mmHg rise in $PaCO_2$	$H^+ + HCO_3^-$ [HCO_3^-] falls by 1 mM for each 10 mmHg fall in $PaCO_2$ [H^+] falls by 8 nmol/L for each 10 mmHg fall in $PaCO_2$	$H^+ + HCO_3^-$ Increased $PaCO_2$	$\rightarrow CO_2 + H_2O$ Increased $PaCO_2$
Example	Hypoventilation	Hyperventilation	Acidosis during controlled ventilation	HCO_3^- administration during controlled ventilation
Chronic compensation	Renal compensation takes $\geq$ 48 h [HCO_3^-] rises by 3–5 mmol/L for each 10 mmHg rise in $PaCO_2$	Renal compensation takes $\geq$48 h [HCO_3^-] falls by 3–5 mmol/L for each 10 mmHg fall in $PaCO_2$	Hyperventilation $PaCO_2$ falls by 1–1.3 mmHg for each 1 m mol/L fall in [HCO_3^-]	Hypoventilation $PaCO_2$ rises by 0.6 mmHg for each 1 mmol/L rise in [HCO_3^-]
Example	Chronic obstructive airway disease	Long-term hyperventilation	Hyperventilation response to acute renal failure, diabetic, ketoacidosis, etc	Limited respiratory compensation to, for example, prolonged vomiting

Figure 4.18 Biochemical features of acid–base disturbances. CO_2, carbon dioxide; H^+, hydrogen; HCO_3^-, hydrogen carbonate; H_2O, water; $PaCO_2$, partial pressure of carbon dioxide.

The most important biological buffers are bicarbonate/CO_2, intracellular phosphate, proteins, and hemoglobin. Of these the most important extracellular system is bicarbonate/CO_2, the activity of which is described by the Henderson–Hasselbalch equation:

$$pH = 6.1 + \log_{10} ([HCO_3^-]/[CO_2])$$

Although the pK_a of this system at 6.1 is some distance from biologic pH, the physiologic importance of the bicarbonate buffer system is due to the high concentration of plasma bicarbonate and the ability of the respiratory and renal systems to adjust the concentrations of CO_2 and hydrogen carbonate (HCO_3^-) in response to changes in plasma pH.

Normal acid–base values are:
- pH = 7.36–7.44
- H^+ = 43–36 nmol/L
- $PaCO_2$ = 35–45 mmHg.

Metabolic status: HCO_3^- = 22–26 mmol/L.

Analysis of acid–base disorders

Modern blood gas analyzers measure pH, $PaCO_2$, and PaO_2. Estimates of metabolic status such as base excess, standard bicarbonate are derived from these values of pH and $PaCO_2$ using assumptions of the normal buffering activity of the body. Since this activity may vary considerably in critically ill patients due to changes in temperature and electrolyte concentrations, it is best to avoid over-reliance on these potentially misleading values and instead to use the following scheme:
- Define the acid–base disturbance from pH or H^+ measurement.
- Examine whether the change in $PaCO_2$ is consistent or incompatible with this primary disturbance (ie, is the disturbance primarily respiratory or metabolic in nature?).
- Decide whether the primary change in pH has been compensated for by a secondary change in $PaCO_2$ or HCO_3^-.

Plotting pH and PaO_2 on acid–base diagrams (which present 95% confidence limits for the observed relationship between pH and PaO_2 in a variety of acid–base disorders) may also aid analysis.

Anion gap and metabolic acidosis

The anion gap measures the difference between the concentration of unmeasured anions (phosphate, lactate, ketones, etc) and cations:

$$Anion\ gap = \{[Na^+] - ([Cl^-] + [HCO_3^-])\}$$

The normal anion gap is 8–12 mmol/L, and can be used to classify metabolic acidosis. With hypoalbuminemia, the 'normal' anion gap decreases by 2.5 for each 1 g/dL fall in albumin below normal (eg, if albumin is 2.0, the 'normal' anion gap is 2.5 × 2.0 = 5 points lower; ie, 3–7 mmol/L).

Metabolic acidosis associated with an increased anion gap

Increased H^+ load combines with HCO_3^-, which is then eliminated as CO_2, thus increasing the anion gap:

$$H^+ + HCO_3^- \rightarrow CO_2 + H_2O$$

Causes include:
- ketoacidosis (diabetic, alcoholic, starvation)
- lactic acidosis
- uremia
- exogenous acids – salicylate, methanol, ethylene glycol.

Metabolic acidosis associated with a normal anion gap

This is caused by a loss of HCO_3^- from the body, with replacement by chloride (Cl^-) and is caused by:
- longstanding diarrhea
- renal tubular acidosis
- hyperchloremic saline (eg, 0.9% saline) resuscitation
- ureterosigmoidostomy
- biliary/pancreatic fistula
- ileostomy
- carbonic anhydrase inhibitors.

Another cause is the addition of acid with Cl^- such as hydrogen chloride, ammonium chloride or lysine hydrochloride.

Chapter 5

Acute renal failure

Imre Noth
University of Chicago, Chicago, IL, USA

Definition

Acute renal failure (ARF) is a reduction in glomerular filtration, with a resulting inability to excrete nitrogenous waste or maintain adequate fluid and acid–base balance, occurring over hours or days. Despite advances in dialysis technology, the mortality of the condition is high even when it is simply the renal manifestation of multiple organ dysfunction syndrome (MODS). However, renal function is potentially recoverable in that a majority of survivors have the potential to return to a dialysis-independent state.

Classification

Prerenal

As many as 70% of patients with ARF are prerenal. Reduced renal perfusion caused by hypovolemia (volume depletion), low cardiac output states, or profound systemic vasodilation (volume redistribution) leads to reductions in glomerular perfusion and urine output. Afferent arteriolar vasodilation and efferent vasoconstriction of the glomerular vessels (mediated by dilating prostaglandins and angiotensin II, respectively) will initially maintain glomerular perfusion pressure at a cost of compromising tubular perfusion. Nonsteroidal anti-inflammatory drugs (NSAIDs) and angiotensin-converting enzyme inhibitors (ACEIs) exacerbate prerenal renal failure by interfering with these compensatory mechanisms. If renal hypoperfusion persists, acute tubular necrosis and established renal failure inevitably develop. The causes of prerenal ARF include the following:

- volume depletion – gastrointestinal loss, excessive diuresis, and salt-wasting nephropathy

- volume redistribution (peripheral vasodilation) – peritonitis, burns, pancreatitis, hypoalbuminemia
- reduced cardiac output – pericardial tamponade, myocardial infarction, acute/chronic valvular disease, cardiomyopathies, arrhythmias.

Intrinsic

Intrinsic cases comprise 25% of all acute renal failure cases. Most cases (90%) of acute intrinsic renal failure are acute tubular necrosis caused by renal ischemia and toxins (including sepsis). The terminal portion of the proximal tubule and the ascending limb of the loop of Henle are most at risk because of their high metabolic activity. Epithelial casts develop, blocking the tubules and further impairing function. Recovery of function is common following acute tubular necrosis, and is brought about by renal parenchymal regeneration. The causes of intrinsic renal failure include:

- renal ischemia
- renal artery/vein thrombosis
- glomerulonephritis
- vasculitides
- hemolytic uremic syndrome/thrombotic thrombocytopenic purpura
- malignant hypertension
- drugs (eg, aminoglycosides, contrast media)
- acute tumor lysis syndrome
- rhabdomyolysis
- allergic interstitial nephritis
- acute pyelonephritis.

Figure 5.1 shows the main differences between the principal types of acute renal failure.

Postrenal

Postrenal cases account for 5% of patients with acute renal failure. Common causes of urinary tract obstruction include:

- prostatic enlargement
- bladder cancer
- ureteric obstruction due to pelvic masses
- bilateral renal calculi.

Diagnosis

While a medical history and physical examination are important in making a diagnosis of acute renal failure, laboratory findings help to define the diagnosis.

Distinction between prenatal and intrinsic ARF		
Variable	Prerenal	Intrinsic
Specific gravity	>1.020	1.010
Urine [Na⁺] (mmol/L)	<10	>20
FE_{Na^+}	<1%	>1%
Casts	Hyaline	Tubular epithelial cells and debris

Figure 5.1 **Distinction between prerenal and intrinsic ARF.** ARF, acute renal failure; FE_{Na^+}, fractional excretion of Na⁺.

Oliguria (urine output < 400 mL/day) may or may not be present. The important laboratory abnormalities include:
- raised urea and creatinine
- hyperkalemia
- metabolic acidosis.

All of the above problems will be exacerbated if they are caused or accompanied by the hypercatabolic state of the systemic inflammatory response syndrome (SIRS) or sepsis. Urinalysis aids the distinction between prerenal and intrinsic renal failure.

The fractional excretion of sodium (FE_{Na^+}) is considered to be the most reliable biochemical laboratory discriminator between prerenal and intrinsic renal failure, and is given by:

$$FE_{Na^+} = \frac{(U_{Na}/Pl_{Na}) \times 100}{(U_{Cr}/Pl_{Cr})}$$

where U_{Na} = urea sodium, Pl_{Na} = plasma sodium, U_{Cr} = urea creatinine, and Pl_{Cr} = plasma creatinine.

The fractional excretion of urea can also be particularly useful in assessing prerenal cases. The urinary bladder must be catheterized and appropriate imaging (ultrasound, CT) performed to exclude obstruction of the renal tract. Autoimmune screens for disorders such as systemic lupus erythematosus (SLE), Wegener's granulomatosis, and Goodpasture syndrome might be indicated, along with renal biopsy if the cause is uncertain.

Treatment
Prerenal renal failure
The aim of treatment is to restore renal perfusion before intrinsic renal failure is established. Recent 'renal rescue' protocols (such as that shown in Figure 5.2) emphasize the need for:
- invasive monitoring

- aggressive fluid resuscitation
- restoration of the patient's systolic blood pressure to a normal level
- avoidance of nephrotoxins
- maintenance of adequate oxygenation, with artificial ventilation if necessary.

Intrinsic renal failure

Renal perfusion should be maintained to eliminate prerenal failure. Measures should be taken to exclude and treat obstructive renal failure. Once intrinsic renal failure is established, general measures can be adopted and these are discussed below.

Fluid balance

Restrict fluid intake to 30 mL/h plus losses (nasogastric, drains, diarrhea, etc) until renal replacement therapy has been instituted.

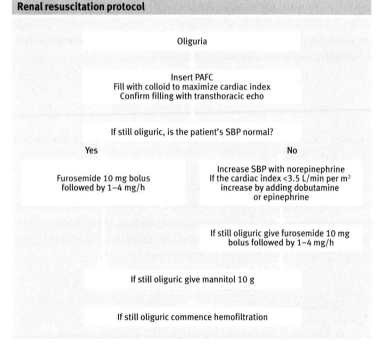

Renal resuscitation protocol

Oliguria

Insert PAFC
Fill with colloid to maximize cardiac index
Confirm filling with transthoracic echo

If still oliguric, is the patient's SBP normal?

Yes

No

Furosemide 10 mg bolus
followed by 1–4 mg/h

Increase SBP with norepinephrine
If the cardiac index <3.5 L/min per m^2
increase by adding dobutamine
or epinephrine

If still oliguric give furosemide 10 mg
bolus followed by 1–4 mg/h

If still oliguric give mannitol 10 g

If still oliguric commence hemofiltration

Figure 5.2 Renal resuscitation protocol. PAFC, pulmonary artery flotation catheter; SBP, systolic blood pressure.

Nutritional support

Adequate nutrition is of considerable importance and should be enteral if at all possible. Caloric requirements may be high in hypercatabolic patients (30–35 kcal/kg daily). Protein requirements are similarly high (1.5–2 g/kg daily), although intake should be restricted to 20–30 g daily until renal replacement therapy has been instituted.

Treatment of hyperkalemia

Treatment is required if EKG changes are present or potassium (K$^+$) levels >6.5 mmol/L. EKG changes signaling hyperkalemia include:

- peaked T waves
- loss of P wave
- broadened QRS complex
- slurring of ST segment into T wave
- sine wave leading to asystole.

If dialysis is not immediately available, the following measures may be used to temporarily redistribute K$^+$ from the plasma or stabilize the myocardium to reduce the risk of arrhythmias:

- Calcium gluconate (10%) 10 mL i.v. over 5 min (or 20 mL if there is hypocalcemia) will reduce the risk of arrhythmias.
- Glucose (50%) 50 mL i.v. will stimulate insulin release, thereby promoting entry of K$^+$ (and glucose) into cells. If hyperglycemia ensues, administer 4–12 units of insulin (routine use of insulin in patients who do not have diabetes carries an unnecessary risk of hypoglycemia).
- Albuterol 5 mg nebulized or 400 mg subcutaneously – β$_2$ agonists reduce plasma K$^+$ by driving it into cells.
- If the patient is acidotic, give sodium bicarbonate (NaHCO$_3$) 50–100 mmol over 1 h but be aware of the usual risks of bicarbonate administration, including fluid overload, worsening of intracellular and cerebrospinal fluid (CSF) acidosis, acute ionized hypocalcemia, and increased carbon dioxide production.
- Eliminate any unnecessary K$^+$ administration in drugs, diet, etc.
- Ion exchange resins (eg, sodium polysytrene solfante [Kayexalate®] 15 g orally or calcium resonium 15 g three times a day orally or as retention enema) provide longer-term control, if dialysis is delayed still further.

Treatment of acidosis

Sodium bicarbonate should be used only when acidosis is severe (pH <7.1), the patient is symptomatic, or if acidosis is associated with acute hyperkalemia. The need for bicarbonate is an indication for dialysis.

Identification and treatment of sepsis

Commence empiric broad-spectrum therapy once cultures have been taken, bearing in mind the potential nephrotoxicity and reduced elimination of many antimicrobials.

Cause-specific therapies

These include:

- mannitol/NaHCO$_3$ in acute rhabdomyolysis
- immunosuppression in SLE, Wegener's granulomatosis, or Goodpasture syndrome
- plasmapheresis, fresh frozen plasma, and prostacyclin in the hemolytic uremic syndrome
- steroids in allergic interstitial nephritis.

Renal replacement therapy is discussed in more detail later in the chapter.

Acute renal support

Indications for acute hemodialysis are as follows:

- fluid overload
- acidosis
- hyperkalemia
- uremia with signs of encephalopathy
- toxins removable by dialysis.

There is no absolute level of plasma urea and creatinine at which therapy should be started. Early dialysis might shorten the course of acute tubular necrosis; excessive dialysis might prolong the maintenance phase via complement activation and hypovolemia. Therapy modes include peritoneal dialysis and hemodialysis.

Peritoneal dialysis

In peritoneal dialysis the peritoneum is used as a dialysis membrane, glucose-based dialysates being delivered in and out of the peritoneal cavity through a catheter inserted in the anterior lower abdominal wall. Advantages include cardiovascular stability without anticoagulation. Disadvantages include respiratory impairment, risk of peritonitis, and hyperglycemia. It is contraindicated in intra-abdominal pathology and recent abdominal surgery. Its popularity has waned with the advent of continuous forms of hemodialysis, and its use in adults is now usually restricted to patients with isolated acute renal failure.

Hemodialysis

All variants of hemodialysis share the need for the following:

- vascular access – this carries the incurrent risks of complications such as infection or thrombosis
- extracorporeal circuit with artificial kidney – activation of complement and circulating neutrophils can lead to cardiorespiratory problems during dialysis, although this is more of a problem with cuprophane membranes than with the newer, more biocompatible membranes (eg, polysulphone and polyamide)
- anticoagulation – heparin is usually used, although prostacyclin can be used in the presence of a coagulopathy.

Potential problems include the following:

- dysequilibrium syndrome – rapid changes in plasma osmolality, leading to cerebral edema, and in some cases intracranial hypertension
- hypovolemia and hypotension
- fluid overload
- hypoxemia – possibly a result of inflammatory reactions initiated within the pulmonary microvasculature
- bleeding and vascular access complications.

Intermittent hemodialysis

Intermittent hemodialysis (Figure 5.3) is usually performed as 4-h sessions daily or on alternate days. It is highly effective, correcting biochemical, metabolic, and acid–base derangements, but it can be impossible to remove sufficient fluid without provoking severe hypotension that might require cardiovascular support. Risks of dysequilibrium and cerebral edema are highest with this method.

Continuous hemodialysis

Continuous hemodialysis (Figure 5.4) is popular in many intensive care units (ICUs) for the treatment of critically ill patients with ARF. It is generally less likely than intermittent hemodialysis to produce hemodynamic instability and therefore is better tolerated by patients with shock or marginal perfusion. Biochemical clearance is not as effective, but fluid removal is easier. A variety of modes is available, which differ according to vascular access, the need for pumps/complex machinery, and effective clearance. Trials comparing continuous with intermittent dialysis approaches have not demonstrated a clear benefit of continuous dialysis with regard to survival from critical illness.

Intermittent hemodialysis

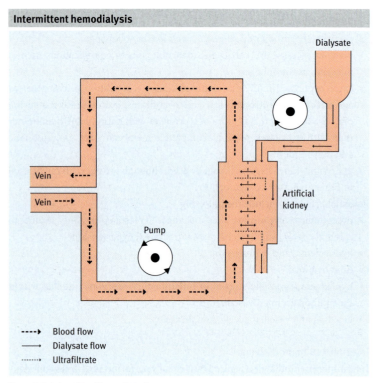

Figure 5.3 Intermittent hemodialysis.

Drugs in renal failure

The dosage regimens of many drugs, commonly used in the ICU, need to be modified in renal failure to avoid accumulation and toxicity. For further information consult the *Physicians Desk Reference,* or the individual drug information sheet. Figure 5.5 shows a list of drugs used in the treatment of renal failure.

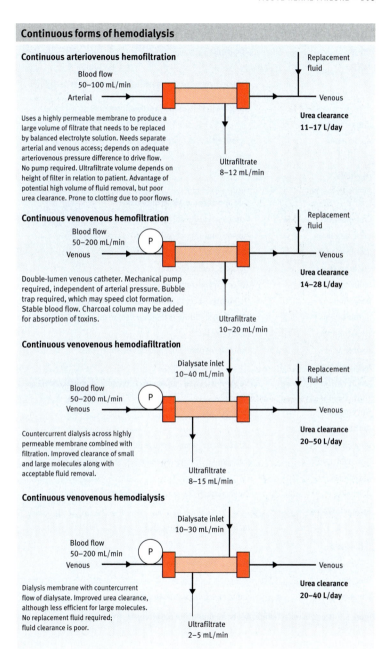

Continuous forms of hemodialysis

Continuous arteriovenous hemofiltration

Blood flow
50–100 mL/min
Arterial

Replacement fluid

Venous

**Urea clearance
11–17 L/day**

Uses a highly permeable membrane to produce a large volume of filtrate that needs to be replaced by balanced electrolyte solution. Needs separate arterial and venous access; depends on adequate arteriovenous pressure difference to drive flow. No pump required. Ultrafiltrate volume depends on height of filter in relation to patient. Advantage of potential high volume of fluid removal, but poor urea clearance. Prone to clotting due to poor flows.

Ultrafiltrate
8–12 mL/min

Continuous venovenous hemofiltration

Blood flow
50–200 mL/min
Venous

P

Replacement fluid

Venous

**Urea clearance
14–28 L/day**

Double-lumen venous catheter. Mechanical pump required, independent of arterial pressure. Bubble trap required, which may speed clot formation. Stable blood flow. Charcoal column may be added for absorption of toxins.

Ultrafiltrate
10–20 mL/min

Continuous venovenous hemodiafiltration

Dialysate inlet
10–40 mL/min

Blood flow
50–200 mL/min
Venous

P

Replacement fluid

Venous

**Urea clearance
20–50 L/day**

Countercurrent dialysis across highly permeable membrane combined with filtration. Improved clearance of small and large molecules along with acceptable fluid removal.

Ultrafiltrate
8–15 mL/min

Continuous venovenous hemodialysis

Dialysate inlet
10–30 mL/min

Blood flow
50–200 mL/min
Venous

P

Venous

**Urea clearance
20–40 L/day**

Dialysis membrane with countercurrent flow of dialysate. Improved urea clearance, although less efficient for large molecules. No replacement fluid required; fluid clearance is poor.

Ultrafiltrate
2–5 mL/min

Figure 5.4 Continuous forms of hemodialysis.

Drugs in renal failure

Drugs	Comments
ACEIs	
	Caution in renovascular disease (can precipitate renal failure)
	Hyperkalemia
	Severe hypotension in hypovolemic patients
Antiarrhythmics	
Amiodarone	Increased risk of thyroid dysfunction
Digoxin	Risk of toxicity increased by hypokalemia; reduce dose
Antibiotics	
Aminoglycosides	Nephrotoxic, ototoxic; monitor plasma levels closely. May be safe and effective given once daily
Ciprofloxacin	Possibly neurotoxic; reduce dose
Cephalosporins	May be nephrotoxic; often require dose reduction
Clarithromycin	Reduce dose
Erythromycin	Ototoxic; reduce dose
Imipenem	Risk of convulsions; reduce dose
Penicillins	Neurotoxic, increased risk of rashes; reduce dose
Sulfonamides	Risk of crystalluria, rashes, and blood disorders
Trimethoprim	Reduce dose
Vancomycin	Ototoxic, nephrotoxic; monitor plasma levels
Antifungals	
Amphotericin	Nephrotoxic; new liposomal or colloidal formulations may be safer
Fluconazole	Reduce dose
Antituberculous drugs	
Ethambutol	Optic nerve damage; reduce dose
Isoniazid	Increased risk of peripheral neuropathy; reduce dose
Antivirals	
Aciclovir	Causes rise in plasma urea; reduce dose
Benzodiazepines	
	Increases cerebral sensitivity
β blockers	
	Adverse effect on renal blood flow; reduce dose
Diuretics	
Furosemide	Rapid injection can cause deafness

Figure 5.5 Drugs in renal failure. ACEIs, angiotensin-converting enzyme inhibitors.

Drugs in renal failure *(Continued)*

Drugs	Comments
Immunosuppressants	
Azathioprine	Reduce dose
Ciclosporin	Nephrotoxic, can cause hyperkalemia; reduce dose
Succinylcholine	Risk of life-threatening hyperkalemia, particularly if plasma potassium levels are elevated
Nondepolarizing drugs	Prolonged paralysis, especially after repeated doses; atracurium and *cis*-atracurium are the safest
NSAIDs	
	Nephrotoxic; sodium/water retention; increased risk of gastrointestinal bleeding
Opioids	Increased cerebral sensitivity
Codeine	Increased/prolonged effect
Dihydrocodeine	Increased/prolonged effect
Dextropropoxyphene	Increased CNS toxicity
Morphine	Delayed elimination
Pethidine	Increased CNS toxicity
Prokinetic drugs	
Metoclopramide	Increased risk of extrapyramidal reactions; reduce dose
Thrombolytics	
Alteplase	Hyperkalemia

Figure 5.5 **Drugs in renal failure** *(Continued)*. CNS, central nervous system; NSAIDs, nonsteroidal anti-inflammatory drugs.

Chapter 6

Neurologic emergencies

Brian Gehlbach
University of Chicago, Chicago, IL, USA

Monitoring of neurological function

Rapid neurologic assessment must include the following:

- assessment of global function (ie, Glasgow Coma Scale score)
- pupillary size, asymmetry, and reactivity
- localizing signs in limbs
- sensory asymmetry
- cardiorespiratory evaluation (the injured brain is exquisitely sensitive to systemic upset, and vice versa).

Glasgow Coma Scale

The Glasgow Coma Scale (GCS) is a semi-quantitative assessment of global neurologic function and is shown in Figure 6.1. In neurotrauma, the post-resuscitation score is more valuable. The modification of the GCS for children (Figure 6.2) is not as reproducible and is less useful; maximum scores for motor and verbal responses are dependent on age and baseline developmental stage.

Pupillary signs

Asymmetry that is greater than 1 mm is abnormal. Figure 6.3 shows the different systems involved in regulating pupillary size.

Causes of pupillary asymmetry

Injury to any aspect of the reflex pathway can result in pupillary asymmetry or unresponsiveness. These include injury to the orbit, globe, and its contents, nerve II, midbrain or brain stem, cervical sympathetic chain, and nerve III. Acute dilation and loss of reactivity to light after a head injury must be assumed to result from a rapidly expanding intracranial space-occupying lesion, and demands

Glasgow Coma Scale

Eye-opening response	Score
Spontaneously	4
To speech	3
To pain	2
None	1
Best motor response	
Obeys commands	6
Localization to painful stimulus	5
Normal flexion to painful stimulus	4
Spastic flexion to painful stimulus	3
Extension to painful stimulus	2
None	1
Best verbal response	
Orientated	5
Confused	4
Inappropriate words	3
Incomprehensible sounds	2
None	1
Total	**15**

Figure 6.1 Glasgow Coma Scale. A severe head injury is defined as a Glasgow Coma Scale (GCS) of 8 or less. Coma is defined as no words, no eye opening, and no response to commands (ie, E1, V2, M5, or worse). Significant deterioration is defined as decrease in GCS of 2 or more.

urgent computed tomography (CT) in a hemodynamically stable patient. Under such circumstances it results from herniation of the uncal component of the temporal lobe through the tentorial hiatus, with a resulting compression of the ipsilateral third nerve.

Argyll Robertson pupils are small, and unreactive to light; however, the accommodation reflex remains intact. Holmes–Adie pupils are large, unreactive, and constrict with convergence. Severe hypotension, drugs, or alcohol are also underlying causes of pupil asymmetry.

Limb signs

When the patient is awake, signs include inequality of movement or strength in the limbs. When the patient is comatose signs include asymmetry of posturing or reflexes, a delayed response, or increasing stimulus for the same response.

Neurologic monitoring of ventilated patient
Clinical monitoring

This can be done by use of the GCS, but it is affected by sedation and the neuromuscular blockade. The pupils are the only definite sign in sedated patients.

Modification of the Glasgow Coma Scale for children	
Eye-opening response	**Score (age at which applicable)**
As for adults	
Best motor response in upper limbs	
Obeys commands	6 (>2 years)
Localizes to pain	5 (<2 years)
Normal flexion to pain	4 (>6 months)
Spastic flexion to pain	3 (<6 months)
Extension to pain	2
None	1
Best verbal response to pain	
Orientated	5 (>5 years)
Words	4 (>12 months)
Vocal sounds	3 (>6 months)
Cries	2 (<6 months)
None	1
Maximum aggregate scores for age	
0–6 months	9
6–12 months	11
1–2 years	13
2–5 years	14
>5 years	15

Figure 6.2 Modification of the Glasgow Coma Scale for children.

Autonomic control of pupillary size		
System	**Efferent pathway**	**Effect**
Parasympathetic	Nerve III	Constriction
Sympathetic	Cervical sympathetic chain	Dilation

Figure 6.3 Autonomic control of pupillary size. Note that parasympathetic influences dominate.

Intracranial pressure monitoring

Ventricular is the gold standard as it allows cerebrospinal fluid (CSF) to be withdrawn; however, there is a higher risk of infection. Parenchymal has a lower infection rate, but recalibration is difficult. Subdural has a lower infection rate, but it is less accurate.

Cerebral oxygenation

Cerebral oxygenation can be done using jugular bulb oximetry. This involves retrograde placement of a catheter in the jugular vein, which allows intermittent or (preferably) continuous measurement of oxygen saturation of the blood leaving the brain ($SjvO_2$):

$$SjvO_2 \propto CBF/CMRO_2$$

where CBF = cerebral blood flow and $CMRO_2$ = cerebral metabolic rate for O_2. If $CMRO_2$ is constant then jugular saturation is dependent on cerebral blood flow.

$SjvO_2$ >90%	Hyperemia
$SjvO_2$ 60–80%	Normal
$SjvO_2$ <50%	Ischemia

Near-infrared spectroscopy is a noninvasive transcranial measure of regional cerebral oxygenation; however, it is unreliable and largely experimental. An indwelling blood–gas electrode is invasive, and measures local tissue pH, and partial pressures of oxygen (PaO_2) and carbon dioxide ($PaCO_2$).

Transcranial Doppler
This is a non-invasive measure of cerebral blood velocities. It is established in the monitoring of vasospasm following spontaneous and traumatic subarachnoid hemorrhage.

Processed electroencephalogram
The processed electroencephalogram (EEG) is of prognostic value following traumatic brain injury. It allows detection of seizure activity in paralyzed patients, and is used to guide therapies designed to reduce cerebral metabolism.

Raised intracranial pressure
Normal intracranial pressure (ICP) is less than 15 mmHg. Factors increasing ICP may also disrupt autoregulation, so that maintenance of adequate cerebral perfusion pressure (CPP) becomes important:

$$CPP = MAP - ICP \text{ (or CVP if greater)}$$

where MAP = mean arterial pressure; CVP = central venous pressure.

Causes

Increased brain tissue mass (eg, due to a tumor, cerebral edema), increased CSF (eg, hydrocephalus), increased cerebral blood volume (eg, hyperemia, drug-induced vasodilation, hypercapnia, coughing and venous hypertension, hematoma) are all causes of raised ICP.

Clinical features

The clinical features of raised ICP vary. Headaches, which are classically worse in the mornings, are common. Other signs include vomiting (typically without nausea), visual disturbances, signs of brain herniation, depressed consciousness level, or coma. Other features include cardiorespiratory changes in preterminal stages, such as Cushing's response of hypertension and bradycardia, and respiratory arrhythmia.

Management

Management of raised ICP depends on the cause and speed of onset. In cases where the cause is a tumor, prophylaxis is administration of dexamethasone and surgery.

Dexamethasone is recommended for the treatment of cerebral edema (for edema associated with tumors); maintenance of CPP >70 mmHg and diuretics (mannitol 0.25–1.0 g/kg every 2–6 h; furosemide may be added) may play a role, but beware of a fall in CPP; use controlled ventilation if respiratory failure occurs. Ventricular drainage is recommended for hydrocephalus.

Brain herniation

Figures 6.4 and 6.5 illustrate herniation syndromes.

Management of acute herniation

Intubation and hyperventilation ($PaCO_2$ 30–35 mmHg or 4–4.7 kPa) can be carried out in order to reduce cerebral blood volume. Mannitol 20% 0.25–1 g/kg ± furosemide can be administered to reduce cerebral water content. Intravenous anesthetic agents (to reduce cerebral metabolic rate and therefore cerebral blood volume) can also be administered. For example, a dose of thiopental 10–20 mg/kg by slow bolus infusion, followed by continuous infusion of up to 5 mg/kg per h to produce burst suppression on EEG, or a dose of etomidate 0.5mg/kg bolus followed by infusion can be given. These agents should be given only by anesthetists with full resuscitation facilities at hand; beware reduction in MAP.

Herniation syndromes

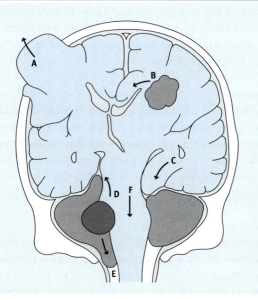

Figure 6.4 Herniation syndromes. A, transcalvarial; **B,** subfalcine; **C,** transtentorial (uncal); **D,** transtentorial ('upward'); **E,** tonsillar; **F,** axial (central or 'coning').

Brain herniation

Type	Neuroanatomic structures at risk	Consequences
Subfalcine	Lateral shift of cingulate gyrus beneath falx, compression of anterior cerebral arteries	Leg weakness
Tentorial		
Lateral (uncal)	Nerve III Posterior cerebral artery Cerebral peduncle	Ptosis, mydriasis, lateral deviation Hemianopsia Hemiparesis
Posterior (tectal)	Quadrigeminal plate	Bilateral ptosis, upward gaze, paralysis
Central (axial)	Reticular formation Corticospinal tracts Midbrain/pons Medulla	Depression of consciousness Decerebrate rigidity Impaired eye reflexes, irregular respiration Hypertension, bradycardia, apnea
Tonsillar	Compression of medulla by cerebellar tonsils	Apnea

Figure 6.5 Brain herniation.

A CT scan to exclude surgical lesions such as a hematoma, tumor, or hydrocephalus should also be carried out. In addition, surgery such as evacuation of a hematoma, lobectomy, subtemporal or posterior fossa decompression, or ventricular drainage can also be performed.

Traumatic brain injury

Primary brain injury occurs on impact and is considered irreversible. Secondary brain injury (Figure 6.6) results from processes initiated by primary insult that occur some time later and may be prevented or ameliorated. Management of traumatic brain injury (TBI) aims to prevent secondary brain injury.

Initial management of traumatic brain injury

- ABC: airway, breathing, circulation
- establish an anatomical diagnosis
- prioritize management
- neurologic assessment and management – post-resuscitation level of consciousness using the GCS (mild: 13–15, moderate: 9–12, severe: ≤8), pupillary function, lateralizing/focal neurology, external examination for depressed, compound, or basal skull fractures.

Indications for a CT scan

Indications for a CT scan are a GCS score that is either less than 9, or less than 15 plus skull fractures, multiple injuries, and persisting for more than 24 h.

Causes of secondary brain injury	
Systemic	**Intracranial**
Hypoxia	Delayed hematoma
Hypotension	Cerebral edema
Hypercapnia	Brain shift/herniation
Hypocapnia	Cerebrovascular injury
Anemia	Vasospasm
Pyrexia	Hydrocephalus
Hypoglycemia	Infection
Hyponatremia	Delayed biochemical cascade of cerebral ischemia
Sepsis	Seizures

Figure 6.6 Causes of secondary brain injury.

Indications for transfer to a neurosurgical center

As with the indications for a CT scan, for the patient to warrant transfer to a neurosurgical center, the patient must have:

- a GSC score that is less than 9
- a 2-point deterioration in GCS
- focal neurologic signs
- a compound skull fracture
- a basal skull fracture
- CT findings of mass lesion or diffuse axonal injury
- a GCS score that is less than 15, persisting for more than 24 h.

Insults leading to secondary brain injury are particularly likely to occur during inter- and intrahospital transfers.

Indications for intubation/ventilation before transfer

Immediately

There are several indications for immediate intubation; these include the patient being in a coma (ie, no eye opening, no words, not obeying commands – E1, V2, M5, or worse) or if there is loss of the protective laryngeal reflexes. Any current or impending respiratory failure, hypoxemia (which is a requirement for high-flow supplemental oxygen), hypercapnia, and excessive work of breathing are all indicators for commencing intubation straight away. Spontaneous hyperventilation (ie, $PaCO_2$ <25 mmHg or <3.3 kPa) and respiratory arrhythmia are also indicators.

Before the start of the transfer

If the patient experiences a significantly deteriorating conscious level (even if not in a coma), a bilateral fractured mandible, copious bleeding into the airway, or seizures, ventilation should be initiated.

Conduct of transfer

The transfer must be conducted according to guidelines agreed locally between the referring hospitals and the neurosurgical unit. The patient must be thoroughly resuscitated and stabilized prior to transfer. In particular, a hypotensive patient must not be transferred until all possible systemic causes have been identified and stabilized. Only in exceptional circumstances should a patient with significant alteration in conscious level not be intubated for transfer. Transfers should be conducted by medical personnel who are familiar with the patient and the treatment to date, and sufficiently experienced in an appropriate specialty and familiar with the pathophysiology and treatment of head injuries. In practice this means an anesthetist who has at least 2 years' experience in the specialty. In addition it is also important that the medical team carrying out the transfer are provided with adequate training in the transport of critically ill patients, personal insurance, and medical indemnity, and accompanied by a suitably trained assistant. The transfer team must also have a means of communication with their base hospital and neurosurgical center (eg, a mobile telephone).

Indications for intracranial pressure monitoring

Patients who have a GCS that is less than 9 should have their ICP monitored, particularly if there is an abnormal CT scan (eg, which shows the presence of a hematoma, contusion, edema, or compressed basal cisterns). When the CT scan is normal, the ICP should be monitored in patients who have two or more of the following:

- age greater than 40 years
- abnormal motor posturing
- systolic BP less than 90 mmHg.

Patients in need of post-operative ventilation, following removal of a mass lesion should also be monitored, as should patients with lesser degrees of head injury who require ventilation for other reasons. Monitoring of ICP enables manipulation of CPP, detection of expanding mass lesions such as a delayed extradural hematoma, and therapeutic withdrawal of CSF (if a ventricular catheter is used).

Secondary management of severe traumatic brain injury
Maintenance of cerebral perfusion pressure

In order to maintain a CPP above 70 mmHg, initially direct therapy towards maintaining or elevating MAP, particularly if compromised by sedation, hemorrhage, diuretics, etc. Expand intravascular volume as necessary with crystalloid, aiming for CVP 5–8 mmHg (or pulmonary artery wedge pressure [PAWP] 12–15 mmHg), with hematocrit 30–35%. If fluid loading alone is inadequate, commence inotropic support using an agent with vasoconstricting properties (eg, norepinephrine). In addition, it is possible to reduce ICP by undertaking the following measures:

- ensure adequate sedation and consider neuromuscular blockade
- check blood gases to exclude hypoxia and hypercapnia
- check position to exclude or minimize venous congestion
- identify and treat seizures
- mannitol 20% 0.5 g/kg may be repeated every 6 h, up to plasma osmolality of about 320 mosmol/L
- furosemide 0.7 mg/kg
- withdrawal of CSF via ventricular catheter

- decompressive craniectomy or lobectomy
- barbiturate coma (thiopental 20 mg/kg + infusion, pentobarbital 3 mg/kg + 1.5 mg/kg per h), to induce burst suppression on processed EEG.

A repeat scan can also help to maintain CPP levels. Indications for a repeat scan are dilating pupil(s) or a refractory intracranial hypertension, particularly if at high risk for evolving surgical pathology, eg, skull fracture, extradural hematoma, contusions, expanding edema, subarachnoid blood, or hydrocephalus.

General measures
General measures of management are given below:

Artificial ventilation
The duration of ventilatory support depends on the nature of the brain injury, other injuries, premorbid state, etc. Causes of prolonged respiratory failure include:
- aspiration
- nosocomial pneumonia (particularly if persisting intracranial hypertension has restricted chest physiotherapy/toilet and necesitated prolonged neuromuscular blockade)
- thoracic trauma
- neurogenic pulmonary edema, and other causes of acute lung injury.

It is important to maintain normocapnia, as prolonged hyperventilation is associated with cerebral ischemia, and adequate oxygenation (with positive end-expiratory pressure [PEEP] if necessary).

Endotracheal intubation may be required for airway protection for some time after weaning from positive-pressure ventilation.

Position
Neutral neck position with slack endotracheal tube (ETT) tapes, and a 15° head-up tilt.

Gastrointestinal protection
Enteral nutrition is preferrable if possible. Sucralfate 1 g every 6 h nasogastrically or ranitidine 50 mg every 8 h can be administered.

Enteral nutrition
Enteral nutrition should be established as soon as possible, using metoclopramide 10 mg every 8 h if necessary to promote gastric emptying. Aim to deliver

100–150% of basal energy requirements. Hyperglycemia should be treated with IV insulin as per sliding scale.

Control of seizures
Benzodiazepine can be administered to terminate seizures. A dose of phenytoin 18 mg/kg over 30 min + 300 mg/day for prevention of further seizures can also be given.

Maintenance of normothermia
Normal body temperature can be sustained by:
- treating the infection
- acetaminophen 325–650 mg every 4–6 h
- diclofenac 150 mg/day
- active cooling (water blanket, cold air convection, etc).

Deep vein thrombosis
Commence deep vein thrombosis (DVT) prophylaxis after 72 h if clotting is normal. Disseminated intravascular coagulation (DIC) may be a result of thromboplastin release and endothelial damage, and should be managed with fresh frozen plasma, cryoprecipitate, and platelets (particularly if contusions or hematomas are present).

Correction of hyponatremia or hypernatremia
See section on disorders of plasma sodium on page 134.

Brain death
Brain death constitutes irreversible cessation of all brain function, and in the US it is considered, medically and legally, to be the death of the individual. Criteria for the diagnosis of brain death have been established by a presidential commission on this topic.

Condition 1: Cerebral functions are absent
The patient must be deeply comatose, with no spontaneous movement and no response to external stimuli such as noise, bright light, or pain. Spinal reflexes may be present, but decorticate or decerebrate posturing cannot be. Rarely, brain-stem lesions may leave the patient paralyzed but with intact cognition ('locked in'), requiring additional studies such as EEG to evaluate cerebral function.

Condition 2: Brain-stem functions are absent

Brain-stem reflexes are examined using the techniques described in Figure 6.7. Respiratory drive is examined by disconnecting the patient from the ventilator for long enough to ensure that the $PaCO_2$ is above the threshold for stimulation of the respiratory center (normally 60 mmHg or 8 kPa). The patient must not be hypotensive during the test:

- Preoxygenate with 100% oxygen for 10 min.
- Disconnect the patient from the ventilator.
- Look for respiratory effort while repeating blood gas analysis to ensure that the $PaCO_2$ threshold has been passed. The $PaCO_2$ will increase at approximately 3 mmHg/min (0.4 kPa).
- Hypoxemia must be prevented during the test – if hypoxemia develops during the above protocol, the following approaches may be used after first restoring oxygenation: one strategy is to hypoventilate the patient with 2–4 breaths/min of 100% oxygen, allowing a more gradual rise in $PaCO_2$. Alternately, hypoxemia may be prevented through the administration of oxygen 6 L/min by passive flow into the trachea.

These guidelines do not address individuals with pre-existing hypercapnia or metabolic alkalosis, in whom a higher threshold for $PaCO_2$ may be required to stimulate breathing.

Condition 3: Cessation of brain function is irreversible

All three of the following must be present to establish this criterion:

1. The cause of the coma is established, and sufficient to explain the loss of brain function. Most causes of loss of brain function can be readily determined though a comprehensive history and physical examination, CT of the brain, basic biochemical laboratories, and drug screening. However, some causes (eg, viral encephalitis or unusual drugs or toxins) may not be obvious, and may require additional testing.

2. There is no possibility of recovery of any brain function. Important causes of reversible loss of brain function include hypothermia (<35°C), drug intoxication, therapeutic barbiturate administration, neuromuscular blockade, and severe hypotension.

3. Cessation of all brain function persists for an appropriate period of observation, and despite (if possible) a trial of therapy. When the precise structural insult is known, 12 h of observation is sufficient. Following a diffuse insult such as cerebral anoxia, 24 h of observation is reasonable. The period of observation must not include time spent hypothermic, severely hypotensive, or intoxicated.

Diagnostic tests for the confirmation of brain death

Tests for brain-stem reflexes	Cranial nerves tested	Comments
The pupils are fixed in diameter and do not respond to sharp changes in the intensity of incident light	II, III	Local trauma may prevent examination of papillary reflexes
There is no corneal reflex	V, VII	Local trauma may prevent examination of corneal reflexes
The cold caloric vestibulo-ocular reflex is absent	III, IV, VI, VIII	Clear access to the tympanic membranes must be established by direct inspection. The reflexes are considered to be absent when no eye movement occurs during or in the 30 s period after the slow irrigation of the external auditory meatus with 20 mL ice-cold water. Local trauma may render this test impossible
No motor responses within the cranial nerve distribution can be elicited by adequate stimulation of any somatic or cranial area	V, VII, IX, XI, XII	Beware of spinal cord injury
There is no gag reflex or reflex response to bronchial stimulation by a suction catheter passed into the trachea	IX, X, XI, XII	

Figure 6.7 Diagnostic tests for the confirmation of brain death.

When the cause of the coma is not clear, or the neurologic evaluation is necessarily incomplete (eg, severe facial trauma), additional testing may be helpful. In selected patients EEG and cerebral blood flow (CBF) studies such as transcranial Doppler ultrasonography or cerebral angiography may be helpful.

Potential pitfalls include trauma to the eyes or ears, chronic respiratory disease affecting blood gas thresholds for apnea testing, locked-in syndrome, brain-stem encephalitis, and unrecognized drug ingestion.

Management of organ donors

Once a potential organ donor has been identified, the regional transplant coordinator should be contacted, but he or she should not be involved in the process of diagnosing brain death or obtaining consent for organ donation. In general, the following features exclude eligibility for organ donation: malignancy (except for primary cerebral, skin, or lip), HIV, hepatitis, intravenous drug abuse, active tuberculosis, and sepsis. However, the regional transplant coordinator should make the determination of eligibility. Once brain death has been declared and the family has consented to organ donation, an aggressive approach to preservation of organ function is crucial.

Investigations of organ donors are shown in Figure 6.8. Additional evaluation specific to each potential organ donation may be required.

Maintenance of homeostasis

Organ perfusion and function should be optimized to maximize chances of continued function in the recipient; it may be compromised by:

- premorbid pathology
- the nature of the injuries
- iatrogenic and nosocomial problems
- consequences of cessation of brain-stem function and loss of medullary control of the cardiovascular system
- fluid and electrolyte imbalance.

General measures

Active warming may be required to maintain a core temperature above 34°C. Continue to prevent or treat infection.

Cardiovascular

Hemodynamic instability often heralds brain death, and hypotension and tachycardia are therefore not uncommon. Hypotension may be further provoked by the diuresis of diabetes insipidus and/or mannitol therapy. A central venous catheter, arterial line, and Foley catheter are often necessary to adequately

Investigations of organ donors	
All donors	Height, weight, blood type, basic chemistries, CBC, PT/PTT, HIV, hepatitis B1 surface antigen, serology for CMV, EBV, *Toxoplasma* spp.
Kidney donors	BUN, creatinine, urinalysis urine culture
Liver donors	Liver function tests Girth around lower costal margin
Heart/heart and lung donors	EKG, chest X-ray, arterial blood gases, chest measurements
Tissue donors	10 mL blood sample

Figure 6.8 **Investigations of organ donors.** BUN, blood urea nitrogen; CBC, complete blood count; CMV, cytomegalovirus; EBV, Epstein–Barr virus; EKG, electrocardiogram; HIV, human immunodeficiency virus; PT, prothrombin time; PTT, partial thromboplastin time.

monitor hemodynamic status. Fluid therapy and vasoactive drug therapy are often necessary to achieve adequate organ perfusion. A systolic blood pressure of 100 mmHg is a reasonable goal. Vasoconstricting agents should be avoided. Supraventricular tachyarrhythmias are common, and can be treated with esmolol. Bradyarrhythmias are unresponsive to atropine, but may be treated with catecholamine infusions. In the event of cardiac arrest, attempts at resuscitation should be made only if organ procurement is imminent (eg, within 15 min).

Respiratory

Maintain oxygenation and normocapnia (note that a reduced production of carbon dioxide may mean that the required minute ventilation is low).

Renal

Diabetes insipidus (DI) occurs in up to 90% of patients and has the following features:

- urine volume > 4 mL/kg per h
- urine osmolality 50–200 mosmol/kg
- plasma osmolality >310 mosmol/kg
- plasma sodium >145 mmol/L.

Other causes of excessive diuresis include mannitol/furosemide therapy for intracranial hypertension, fluid loading, and dopamine infusion, but they can be distinguished from DI by the above features. Hypovolemia is likely without prompt replacement of hourly losses using 5% dextrose with electrolyte supplementation as guided by regular measurement of plasma electrolytes. Deamino-D-arginine vasopressin (DDAVP or desmopressin) 0.5–2.0 mg i.v. every 8–12 h should be given when losses persist for 2 h or more. In the absence of DI maintain urine output of at least 1 mL/kg per h with colloid ± dopamine and furosemide as necessary.

Hematology

Aim for hematocrit of 25–35%. Correct coagulopathies as necessary.

Temperature

Maintain a temperature of 35 °C or more with warmed humidified gases, surface heating, and warmed fluids.

Intraoperative management

Continue supportive therapies and monitoring as discussed above. Use volatile agents such as isoflurane to control hemodynamic changes. Neuromuscular blockade (eg, pancuronium 0.15 mg/kg) is required to prevent spinal reflexes and improve surgical access. Be prepared to give heparin and steroids at the request of the surgical team. Stop monitoring once the major vessels are cross-clamped; stop intermittent positive-pressure ventilation once the trachea has been sectioned.

Guillain–Barré syndrome

Guillain–Barré syndrome is a demyelinating polyneuropathy affecting mainly the peripheral and autonomic nervous systems. It is more common in adults and may be preceded by acute viral illness 1–4 weeks before onset. Other predisposing factors include surgery, pregnancy, malignancy, and acute sero-conversion to HIV.

Clinical features

Guillain–Barré syndrome progresses over days, generally reaching a peak at day 14. It is accompanied by a slowly ascending and usually symmetrical weakness, and 20% of patients show involvement of facial, bulbar, ocular, and respiratory muscles. Afferent effects include areflexia, paresthesia, and distal sensory loss. Autonomic features include dysrhythmias, postural hypotension, and paralytic ileus.

Diagnosis

A diagnosis is made by looking at the clinical features, demyelinating block on nerve conduction studies, and elevated CSF protein, which may be normal in the first few days of illness, but once elevated remains high for several months.

Differential diagnoses

A differential diagnosis may include poliomyelitis, botulism, and primary muscle disease.

Management
Supportive

Several supportive measures can be carried out and these are outlined below.

General

General supportive measures include the prevention of nosocomial and iatro-genic problems (eg, infection), high-quality nursing, and physiotherapy, with frequent turning and passive limb movements. Neuropathic pain is common, and nonsteroidal anti-inflammatory drugs, opioids, or carbamazepine may be required.

Respiratory

Measure vital capacity (VC) daily; consider intubation or ventilation if VC is less than 12 mL/kg or if the bulbar muscles are involved. Use ventilatory modes that encourage spontaneous ventilatory effort (eg, synchronized intermittent mandatory ventilation with pressure support) if possible. Autonomic neuropathy may exaggerate the hemodynamic effects of positive-pressure ventilation (particularly PEEP). In prolonged cases, tracheostomy may be required.

Cardiovascular

Hemodynamic instability resulting from autonomic neuropathy should be managed with appropriate fluid therapy, avoidance of antihypertensive medication, gentle changes in posture, etc. Other causes such as sepsis and myocardial ischemia should be considered. DVT prophylaxis with antiembolic stockings and low-dose subcutaneous heparin is recommended.

Gastrointestinal

Nutrition should be enteral if possible. In the absence of enteral nutrition use sucralfate to protect gastric mucosa. Percutaneous gastrostomy may be needed in prolonged cases.

Specific

High-dose gamma-globulin therapy or plasmapheresis is equally effective when given early (within 7 days of onset) in reducing the severity and duration of the disease. Steroids have no proven benefit.

Complications

Complications include infection, pulmonary embolus, and nerve palsies.

Prognosis

Recovery takes 4 weeks to 1 year, and is incomplete in 10–15% of cases. A slower onset is associated with prolonged recovery. Mortality rates are 1–2%.

Myasthenia gravis

This is an autoimmune disease mediated by IgG antibodies against acetylcholine (ACh) receptors at the motor endplate. It is characterized by weakness and exaggerated fatiguability with sustained effort that improves with rest, and is associated with other autoimmune diseases such as hypothyroidism, rheumatoid arthritis, pernicious anemia, and systemic lupus erythematosus (SLE).

Clinical features

These include:

- ocular – diplopia, ptosis
- bulbar – dysphagia, dysarthria
- limb/trunk – asymmetrical fatigue, respiratory embarassment (exacerbated by aspiration).

Acute deterioration may be precipitated by:

- inadequate or excessive anticholinesterase therapy
- other drugs (eg, anesthetic agents, muscle relaxants, aminoglycoside antibiotics)
- infection
- surgery
- pregnancy
- electrolyte imbalance
- psychological stress.

It is expected that 10–20% of patients will have a thymoma (25% are malignant), and up to 80% will improve following thymectomy. The term 'myasthenic crisis' is reserved for patients with impending respiratory failure.

Diagnosis

Diagnosis can be made by initially noting the clinical features. An edrophonium test (must have resuscitation facilities available) can also be carried out:

- atropine 0.6 mg + edrophonium 2 mg i.v.
- if no response after 45 s, edrophonium 8 mg
- a rapid improvement lasting 2–3 min indicates a positive result.

Electromyogram (EMG) studies can also be undertaken; there is a decremental evoked motor response to repetitive motor nerve stimulation at low rates (3 Hz). An ACh receptor antibody assay (antibodies present in 90% of cases) is also useful.

Differential diagnoses

- botulism
- Lambert–Eaton myasthenic syndrome
- organophosphate poisoning.

Management of myasthenic crisis

Supportive

Supportive measures include the following:

- intubate if bulbar involvement or aspiration risk

- ventilate if VC is less than 12 mL/kg, maximum expiratory pressure (MEP) less than 40 cmH$_2$O
- avoid hypokalemia, hypocalcemia, hypermagnesemia
- enteral feeding
- anti-thromboembolic stockings, low-dose heparin
- intensive nursing and physiotherapy support.

Specific

Specific measures include anticholinesterase, and immunosuppressive therapy:

- Anticholinesterase therapy – pyridostigmine 60–120 mg every 6 h orally (IV dose is 1/30th oral dose) or neostigmine 15–30 mg every 4 h orally. Treat muscarinic side effects (diarrhea, abdominal cramps, etc) with glycopyr-rolate 1 mg every 8 h as required.
- Immunosuppressive therapy – pulsed methylprednisolone 2 g over 12 h every 5 days plus prednisolone 20–100 mg/day; azathioprine 1–3 mg/kg per day or cyclophosphamide 2 mg/kg per day; plasmapheresis: 5 single-volume exchanges over 10–14 days; improvement within days or weeks. Anticholinesterase therapy is usually withheld during plasmapheresis.

Complications

Possible complications may include nosocomial or aspiration pneumonia, sepsis, thromboembolism, or a cholinergic crisis (ie, where excessive ACh levels precipitate depolarizing blockade of receptors). The last should be suspected if symptoms worsen following the edrophonium test, and is best managed by reducing anticholinesterase therapy.

Lambert–Eaton myasthenic syndrome

The Lambert–Eaton myasthenic syndrome (LEMS) is a disorder of neuromus-cular transmission secondary to IgG-mediated impairment of presynaptic, voltage-sensitive calcium channels. Clinical features include muscle weakness (proximal worse than distal, typically sparing bulbar muscles) and autonomic symptoms such as dry mouth and impotence. It is associated with malignancy, SLE, and other autoimmune disorders. IgG antibodies may be detected in 50% of patients. Treatments include:

- anticholinesterases – of limited effectiveness
- immunosuppression
- immunoglobulin
- 3,4-diaminopyridine
- guanidine.

Tetanus

Contamination of a wound by *Clostridium tetani* spores from animal feces or soil causes local infection. Germination releases the exotoxins tetanospasmin and tetanolysin. Tetanospasmin migrates via alpha and gamma motor fibers to the ventral horns of the spinal cord or cranial nerve nuclei and also systemically via the lymphatics in major infections. Presynaptic accumulation prevents neurotransmitter release from inhibitory neurons, explaining the clinical features. The incubation period varies from days to months, although it is generally less than 2 weeks, and shorter in the cephalic form of the disease (shorter migration distance).

Clinical features

Stiffness progressing to rigidity and spasm (Figure 6.9). Autonomic involvement leads to tachycardia, hypo- and hypertensive crises, fever, and sweating.

Diagnosis

Diagnosis is made by observation of clinical features and by a wound Gram stain and culture, which is positive in 30% of cases.

Differential diagnoses

- neuroleptic acute dystonic reaction
- Bell's palsy
- strychnine poisoning
- meningitis
- electrolyte disorders (eg, hypocalcemia)
- rabies.

Management

Treatment of tetanus requires good airway management (eg, in cases of dysphagia or generalized rigidity, intubation is necessary), and where there is

Effects of tetanus	
Muscle involved	**Clinical effect**
Masseter	Dysphagia, trismus
Facial	Risus sardonicus
Vertebral/antigravity	Opisthotonus
Respiratory	Apnea
Perineal	Urinary retention

Figure 6.9 Effects of tetanus.

respiratory compromise intubation, sedation (± paralysis), and ventilation are needed. Benzodiazepine and an opioid can be used to treat muscle spasms and pain; dantrolene may be helpful. For hemodynamic management administer magnesium 70 mg/kg followed by 1–3 g/h (aiming for plasma level of 2.5–4 mmol/L, checking every 4 h). Excise the wound with a 2-cm margin. Human tetanus immunoglobulin (hTIG) is given (intrathecal hTIG 250 IU in cerebral tetanus). Benzylpenicillin 1–3 MU is given every 6 h for 10 days. Nurse in a quiet environment, avoiding any unnecessary stimulation, as this can provoke muscular and autonomic spasms. Active immunization should be completed before leaving hospital.

Complications
Apnea and cardiac arrest are likely complications, as are rhabdomyolysis and acute renal failure, vertebral and long bone fractures, nosocomial infections, and pulmonary embolism.

Prognosis
The mortality rate is between 10% and 20%, and is worse in craniofacial cases, and cases that evolve rapidly.

Botulism

Clostridium botulinum is an anaerobic Gram-positive bacillus with spores in soil or food that may germinate and produce neurotoxins – predominantly A, B, and E in humans; these induce neuromuscular blockade by reducing ACh release. These neurotoxins are destroyed by heating them for more than 120°C for 20 min. Three types of botulism are recognized:

1. Food-borne – following ingestion of canned vegetables or meat (fruit is too acidic)
2. Infantile – induced by toxin produced *in vivo*, associated with honey
3. Wound related.

Clinical features
Clinical features develop approximately 18 h after ingestion and include the following:
- nausea, vomiting, constipation, dry mouth, thirst
- urinary retention
- laryngeal, pharyngeal paralysis
- ptosis and strabismus due to lateral rectus weakness
- pupils that are fixed and either dilated or mid-sized

- descending, symmetrical paralysis
- vertigo.

The level of consciousness is unaffected.

Diagnosis

Clinical features, and identifying the toxin in feces, serum, and food samples, indicate a clear diagnosis. EMG shows small evoked action potentials, increasing with repeated stimulation (in contrast to myasthenia gravis).

Differential diagnoses

- Guillain–Barré syndrome
- myasthenia gravis
- LEMS.

Management
Supportive

Monitor respiratory function (eg, vital capacity, blood gases) as 30% of cases require ventilation. It is also important to prevent complications associated with paralysis such as pressure sores, nerve palsies, etc. Débride the wound if appropriate.

Specific

Gastric lavage and enemas can be carried out to remove unabsorbed neurotoxin. Equine serum botulism antitoxin is used for adults and for children over 1 year of age; skin test the antitoxin before administration. Human-derived botulinum antitoxin is used for infants less than 1 year of age who are diagnosed with infant botulism. Botulism immunoglobulin is also available for use in infant botulism. In adults, administer penicillin 3 MU every 4 h. Guanidine (to increase ACh release) may also be considered.

Prognosis

The mortality rate is 15–50% due to respiratory failure; the infantile variant has a 2% mortality rate. Chronic muscle weakness may persist.

Epilepsy and status epilepticus
Etiology of seizures
1. Metabolic:
   (a) congenital
   (b) acquired:
      - hypoglycemia

- hyperglycemia
- hypoxia
- hypocalcemia
- hyponatremia
- uremia
- toxins
- drugs (withdrawal or intoxication, eg, alcohol, 'angel dust', cocaine).

2. Structural:
   (a) Gliotic scars:
   - temporal lobe sclerosis
   - post-traumatic
   - post-infarction
   - post-infection
   (b) congenital malformations
   (c) vascular malformations (arteriovenous malformation, cavernoma)
   (d) tumor.

3. Infectious:
   (a) systemic (febrile convulsion, hyperthermia).
   (b) intracranial:
   - meningitis
   - encephalitis
   - abscess.

Status epilepticus

Status epilepticus is a condition in which epileptic events persist for more than 30 min, or when the rate of recurrent events is such that the return of consciousness is not possible (Figure 6.10). The most common form is tonic–clonic status epilepticus, although other types are recognized (Figure 6.11). Causes include the following:

- poor antiepileptic drug compliance
- alcohol abuse or withdrawal
- drug toxicity, abuse, or withdrawal
- metabolic disorders
- cerebrovascular disease
- trauma
- infection/ tumours of the central nervous system (CNS).

Pseudostatus is characterized by resistance to passive eye opening, persistence of conjunctival reflex, downgoing plantars, and absence of cyanosis.

Stages of status epilepticus

Stage	Description
Premonitionary	Gradual increase in seizure frequency; this stage may last several hours
Early status 0–30 min	Increased brain metabolism matched by increase in cerebral blood flow and energy supply
Established status 30–120 min	Continued status despite initial treatment; balance between brain energy supply and demand deteriorating
Refractory status >120 min	Continued seizures despite aggressive therapy; high morbidity and mortality

Figure 6.10 Stages of status epilepticus.

Classification of epilepsy

Classification	Symptom
Tonic–clonic	Unconsciousness Generalized tonic contractions progressing to clonic seizure
Generalized absence (petit mal)	Brief episode of unconsciousness. Little or no motor accompaniment
Simple partial seizure	Focal epileptic phenomenon with no loss of consciousness, unless it develops into a generalized seizure
Complex partial seizure	Abnormal behavior, sensations, mood, etc. May develop into a generalized convulsion. Usually arises from temporal lobe
Atonic (akinetic) seizure	Generalized loss of muscle tone. Patient falls down. No loss of consciousness
Myoclonic seizures	Sudden uncontrollable jerks associated with epileptiform electroencephalogram discharges

Figure 6.11 Classification of epilepsy.

Management of status epilepticus

The aims of treatment are to maintain oxygenation and stop seizures within 30 min to prevent brain damage (after 30 min, physiological mechanisms for matching CBF to the increased rate of cerebral metabolism become exhausted and ischemic brain injury becomes more likely).

Supportive treatment

Supportive treatment follows the ABC method, as outlined below:

- **A**irway: oropharyngeal airway or ETT
- **B**reathing: oxygen by facemask and reservoir; may require mechanical ventilation to maintain oxygenation and normocapnia
- **C**irculation: IV access, 0.9% saline infusion + 50 mL 50% dextrose + 250 mg thiamine.

Specific treatment

See Figure 6.12, which shows specific treatments for status epilepticus.

Specific treatment of status epilepticus

Stage	General measures	Anti-seizure medication	Dose and route of administration
Premonitionary	Close neurologic observation; give oxygen and establish IV access	Lorazepam	4 mg i.v. bolus (max . 2 mg/min)
		Diazepam	10 mg IV bolus (max. 5 mg/min)
		Paraldehyde	5–10 mL in 5–10 mL of water/oil per rectum
Early status	SaO_2, EKG, and BP monitoring; check blood glucose, urea and electrolytes, arterial blood gases	*First line* Lorazepam Diazepam *Second line* Fosphenytoin	4–8 mg IV bolus 10–20 mg IV bolus Load 18 phenytoin equivalents/kg i.v. at a rate of 150 mg/min
		Paraldehyde	50–100 mL/h of 4% solution i.v.
		Lidocaine	IV bolus followed by infusion
Established status (30–120 min)	Administer thiamine 100 mg i.v. and 50 mL 50% dextrose; treat acidosis; consider anesthesia, phenobarbital, intubation, and ventilation.	*First line* Fosphenytoin	Load as above if not already administered 10–20 mg/kg i.v. <100 mg/min
		Second line Diazepam Midazolam Paraldehyde	IV infusion IV infusion IV infusion
Refractory status (>120 min)	Anesthesia and ventilation on intensive care unit with invasive arterial and CVP monitoring; paralysis will attenuate the systemic effects of status, but processed EEG monitoring will be required. Pressor therapy may be required to support circulation	*First line* Pentobarbital Propofol	6–8 mg/kg over 1 h followed by 1–5 mg/ kg per h 1–2 mg/kg bolus followed by 3–6 mg/ kg per h
		Second line Isoflurane	Via ventilator

Figure 6.12 Specific treatment of status epilepticus. BP, blood pressure; CVP, central venous pressure; EEG, electroencephalograpy; EKG, electrocardiogram; IV, intravenous; SaO_2, arterial oxygen saturation. Note that full resuscitative facilities and adequate monitoring should be available.

Complications

Likely complications are an ischemic brain injury or systemic. Examples of systemic problems are:

- tissue hypoxia and acidosis
- rhabdomyolysis
- acute tubular necrosis
- disseminated intravascular coagulation
- acute hepatitis
- hypoglycemia
- hyperpyrexia
- tracheobronchial hypersecretion
- elevated growth hormone, prolactin, glucagon.

Investigations

Tests that can be carried out include:

- blood – glucose, urea and electrolytes, acid–base and blood gases, liver function tests, clotting, alcohol, antiepileptic drug levels, and toxicology screen
- EEG
- MRI/CT
- lumbar puncture.

Disorders of plasma sodium

Plasma sodium, as the principal component of plasma osmolality, is a major determinant of fluid shifts across the blood–brain barrier. Disorders of plasma sodium are common in neurologic and neurosurgical disease and are an important reversible cause of neurologic deficit. Figure 6.13 shows some of the clinical features and treatment of plasma sodium disorders.

Diabetes insipidus

DI is a failure to produce concentrated urine, despite a rising plasma osmolality, associated with a lack of production of antidiuretic hormone (ADH) (neurogenic) or a lack of renal response to ADH (nephrogenic). For causes of DI see Figure 6.14.

Syndrome of inappropriate antidiuretic hormone secretion

The syndrome of inappropriate ADH secretion (SIADH) is marked by excessive water retention and (dilutional) hyponatremia associated with the continued

Clinical features and treatment of disorders of plasma sodium

Parameter	SIADH	Cerebral salt wasting	Diabetes insipidus
Blood pressure	Normal	Low/ postural hypotension	Low/ normal
Heart rate	Low/ normal	Resting/postural tachycardia	Normal/ increased
Body weight (total body water)	Normal/ increased	Low	Low/ normal
Urea, creatinine	Low/ normal	Normal/ high	Normal/ high
Blood			
Volume (CVP)	Increased	Low	Low
Hematocrit	Low	High	High
Na$^+$	<135 mM	<135 mM	>145 mM
Osmolality	<280 mOsm	<280 mOsm	>295 mOsm
Urine			
Volume	Low/normal	Low/normal	Increased
Specific gravity	>1.010	>1.010	<1.004
Na$^+$	>25 mM	>25 mM	<25 mM
24-hour secretion of Na$^+$	>30 mmol	>30 mmol	<30 mmol
Osmolality	Frequently >Serum osmolality	>Serum osmolality	<Serum osmolality
Treatment			
Na$^+$	Supplement with 0.9% NaCl or, in severe cases, 200–400 mL 3% NaCl at 4 mL/hour; avoid rises in serum Na$^+$ >10 mM/day	Supplement with 0.9–3% NaCl, depending upon urgency of need to correct	Others
Water	Restrict to 800–1000 mL/day	Supplement	Supplement
Others	Desmocycline 300 mg q 6 hours

Furosemide if overloaded
Consider vasopressin receptor antagonists | | DDAVP 1–4 mg IV Chlorpropamide 200–500 mg/day Carbamazepine 400–600 mg/day Chlorthalidone 100 mg twice a day (nephrogenic DI) |

Figure 6.13 Clinical features and treatment of disorders of plasma sodium.
CVP, central venous pressure; DDAVP, deamino-D-arginine vasopressin; DI, diabetes insipidus; Na$^+$, sodium; NaCl, sodium chloride; SIADH, syndrome of inappropriate antidiuretic hormone secretion.

Causes of diabetes insipidus	
Familial	Autosomal dominant and recessive variants
Traumatic	Pituitary surgery (usually transient), head injury
Inflammatory	Meningitis, encephalitis, tuberculosis, sarcoidosis, histiocytosis, Wegener's granulomatosis
Neoplastic	Lymphoma, leukemia, metastatic bronchial carcinoma, primary tumors in the vicinity of pituitary or hypothalamus
Vascular	Sheehan syndrome, anterior communicating artery aneurysm, massive subarachnoid hemorrhage, metastatic carcinoma

Figure 6.14 Causes of diabetes insipidus.

secretion of ADH despite plasma hypo-osmolality. Causes of SIADH include the following:

1. Central hypersecretion of ADH:
   (a) hypothalamic disorders (eg, trauma, surgery, metabolic encephalopathy, subarachnoid hemorrhage, acute intermittent porphyria, myxedema, vascular lesions)
   (b) suprahypothalamic disorders (eg, cerebral infarction, subdural hematoma, meningitis).
2. Peripheral hypersecretion of ADH:
   (a) pulmonary pathology (eg, infection, bronchial carcinoma)
   (b) recumbent posture.
3. Drugs: vincristine, chlorpropamide, cyclophosphamide, chlorothiazide, carbamazepine, chlorpromazine.

Cerebral salt wasting

This is plasma hyponatremia associated with a persistent urinary loss of sodium, distinguished from SIADH by a decreased plasma volume (in contrast to the expanded plasma volume of SIADH). It is associated with subarachnoid hemorrhage, head injury, and cerebral infarction.

Management of hyponatremia

Correction must not exceed 20 mol/L per 48 h and generally at a rate of no more than 0.5 mmol/L per h.

Hypernatremia must also be avoided so it is best to aim for about 130 mmol/L. In deciding the right amount of sodium (Na^+), the following is a useful guide:

- Na^+ (mmol) $= 0.6 \times$ weight (kg) $\times$ (target $[Na^+]$ – plasma $[Na^+]$)
- quantitate losses from urine, etc.

It is important to frequently reassess plasma and urine for sodium.

Bacterial meningitis

Bacterial meningitis is an inflammation of the meningeal coverings of the brain and spinal cord caused by a variety of organisms. Features in children may be subtle and rapidly progressive. Figures 6.15–6.17 show the properties of normal CSF and the variation and abnormalities as a result of bacterial meningitis.

Clinical features

Headache, neck stiffness, a deteriorating level of consciousness, and systemic sepsis are all indicators for bacterial meningitis.

Diagnosis

Diagnosis is by clinical assessment, blood cultures, and CSF microscopy and culture.

Properties of normal lumbar cerebrospinal fluid	
Cl⁻	110–129 mmol/L
Cells	<5 WBCs/mm³
Glucose	48–86 mmol/L
Osmolality	306 mosmol/kg
pH	7.33–7.37
Pressure	10–15 cmH$_2$O CSF (lateral position)
Production	0.4 mL/min
Protein	
Albumin:globulin	2:1 (infants 1:1)
IgG	10–12% of total protein
Total	15–45 mg/L
Specific gravity	1.0062–1.0082
Volume	140 mL

Figure 6.15 **Properties of normal lumbar cerebrospinal fluid.** Cl⁻, chloride; CSF, cerebrospinal fluid; IgG, immunoglobulin G; WBC, white blood cell.

Variations in cerebrospinal fluid			
	Cisterna	Lumbar	Ventricle
Glucose (mmol/L)	72	61	80
Protein (mg/L)	20	40	10

Figure 6.16 **Variations in cerebrospinal fluid.**

Abnormalities of cerebrospinal fluid

Bloodstained	>500:1 RBC:WBC may be normal (ie, traumatic tap)
Reduced Cl⁻	Tuberculous meningitis
Reduced glucose	Bacterial meningitis
Raised IgG	Disseminated sclerosis, Guillain–Barré syndrome, carcinomatosis
Raised protein	Bacterial meningitis, Froin syndrome
Turbidity	>400 WBCs/mm³ >200 RBCs/mm³
Raised WBC count	
Eosinophils	Parasite infection, TB, syphilis, fungi, lymphoma, Hodgkin's disease, disseminated sclerosis
Mononuclear cells	Viral/TB meningitis, acute demyelination
Polymorphonuclear cells	Bacterial meningitis (or early viral)
Xanthochromia	Breakdown of RBCs – old hemorrhage

Figure 6.17 Abnormalities of cerebrospinal fluid. Cl⁻, chloride; IgG, immunoglobulin G; RBC, red blood cell; TB, tuberculosis; WBC, white blood cell.

Empiric antibiotic therapy for bacterial meningitis

Immune status	Antibiotic	Likely pathogens
Immunocompetent		
<1 month	Ampicillin + cefotaxime or ampicillin plus an aminoglycoside	*Streptococcus agalactiae* *Escherichia coli* *Listeria monocytogenes* *Klebsiella* spp.
1–23 months	Vancomycin plus a third-generation cephalosporin	*Streptococcus pneumoniae* *Neisseria meningitidis* *Streptococcus agalactiae* *Haemophilus influenzae* *Escherichia coli*
2–50 years	Vancomycin plus a third-generation cephalosporin	*Neisseria meningitidis* *Streptococcus pneumoniae*
>50 years	Vancomycin plus ampicillin plus a third-generation cephalosporin	*Streptococcus pneumoniae* *Neisseria meningitidis* *Listeria monocytogenes* Gram-negative bacilli
Immunocompromised	Variable	Numerous
Head trauma, ventricular shunt, neurosurgery	Vancomycin + ceftazidime	*Staphylococcus* spp. Gram-negative bacilli *Streptococcus pneumoniae*

Figure 6.18 Empiric antibiotic therapy for bacterial meningitis.

Specific therapy

Figures 6.18 and 6.19 show empiric and specific therapies available for the treatment of bacterial meningitis. The use of adjunctive dexamethasone is recommended for infants and children with suspected *Haemophilus influenza* type b meningitis and for adults with suspected or proven pneumococcal meningitis.

Specific therapy for bacterial meningitis[†]		
Microbiology	**Antibiotics**	**Duration**
Gram stain		
Positive cocci	Vancomycin + cefotaxime	
Negative cocci	Penicillin 0.3 MU/kg per day to a maximum of 24 MU/kg per day	
Positive bacilli	Ampicillin + gentamicin (1.5 mg/kg)	
Negative bacilli	Head trauma: cefotaxime Shunts: ceftazidime	
Culture		
S. pneumoniae	Cefotaxime or ceftriaxone	14 days
H. influenzae	Cefotaxime or ciprofloxacin	7 days
N. meningitidis	Penicillin	7 days
L. monocytogenes	Ampicillin + gentamicin	14–21 days
S. agalactiae	Penicillin	
Enterobacteriaceae	Cefotaxime + gentamicin	
Pseudomonas aeruginosa, Acinetobacter spp.	Ceftazidime + gentamicin, ciprofloxacin	

Figure 6.19 Specific therapy for bacterial meningitis. [†]Vancomycin should be added in regions with penicillin- or cephalosporin-resistant pneumococci pending sensitivities.

Chapter 7

The endocrine system

John Kress
University of Chicago, Chicago, IL, USA

In the setting of critical illness, endocrine dysfunction may be the primary problem or it may develop as a consequence of another illness. In the latter event, such endocrine dysfunction is often difficult to detect clinically, and a high index of suspicion is therefore necessary.

Diabetic ketoacidosis

Insulin is an important anabolic hormone, having crucial effects on the intermediate metabolism of protein, lipid, and carbohydrate. Its effects are opposed by counterregulatory hormones such as glucocorticoids, glucagon, catecholamines, growth hormone, and human chorionic gonadotropin.

Causes of diabetic ketoacidosis

The principal causes of diabetic ketoacidosis (DKA) are absolute and relative insulin deficiency (Figure 7.1):

- Absolute insulin deficiency: new-onset type 1 diabetes mellitus or interruption of insulin treatment is the main cause of absolute insulin deficiency.
- Relative insulin deficiency: can be caused by an acute illness (eg, when the stress response associated with the illness promotes increased levels of counterregulatory hormones), intercurrent endocrine disorders (eg, hyperthyroidism and pheochromocytoma), drugs (eg, steroids), and pregnancy.

Clinical features

The clinical features of DKA are:

- dehydration and hypotension
- tachypnea, air hunger

Pathophysiology of diabetic ketoacidosis

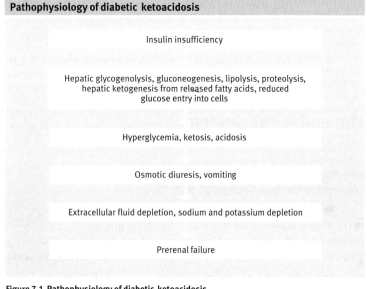

Figure 7.1 Pathophysiology of diabetic ketoacidosis.

- nausea and vomiting
- abdominal pain (often confused with acute abdomen)
- confusion, lowered conscious level
- breath, which smells of acetone.

Laboratory features

The laboratory findings associated with DKA are:
- hyperglycemia
- ketonuria/ketonemia
- metabolic acidosis ± secondary respiratory alkalosis
- hypernatremia and hyperkalemia (despite total body depletion)
- hypertriglyceridemia
- uremia
- leukocytosis, hemoconcentration.

Management

Monitoring

Patients with DKA are best cared for in an intensive care unit (ICU) due to the need for:

- continuous EKG and arterial oxygen saturation (SaO_2)

- hourly urine output
- neurologic observations
- hourly blood sugar, acid–base, and serum potassium
- complete blood count, urea and electrolytes, plasma osmolality, calcium, phosphate, and magnesium on admission, and as indicated thereafter.

Fluid and electrolyte resuscitation

Establish two wide-bore peripheral venous lines – the volume depletion may exceed 10 L. Various regimens are suggested, one approach being to administer sodium chloride (NaCl):

- 2 L 0.9% NaCl over 30 min
- 1 L 0.9% NaCl over 1 h
- 1 L 0.9% NaCl over 2 h
- 1 L 0.9% NaCl over 4 h
- 1 L 0.9% NaCl over 6 h.

This can then be changed to 5–10% dextrose when the blood glucose falls below 180 mg/dL. Regular reassessment of fluid status is vital and is indicated by improving clinical and metabolic status, adequate urine output, and improving biochemistry.

Although the patient may be hypernatremic and hyperkalemic on admission, electrolyte depletion may be profound (Na^+ 8 mmol/kg, K^+ 4 mmol/kg). If the plasma Na^+ exceeds 155 mmol/L after the first hour of resuscitation change to 0.45% NaCl, monitoring plasma Na^+ hourly. After urine flow is established, add potassium to the IV infusion according to the regimen in Figure 7.2.

Hypophosphatemia may also be seen, and should be treated with potassium phosphate at 5 mmol/h.

Insulin therapy

The initial aim is to inhibit ketogenesis, which is achieved with modest doses of insulin. Rapid reductions in blood glucose should be avoided, aiming for a fall

Regimen for addition of potassium to intravenous infusion	
Plasma potassium (mmol/L)	Potassium chloride (mmol)
> 5	0
4–5	13
3–4	26
< 3	39

Figure 7.2 Regimen for addition of potassium to intravenous infusion.

of 90 mg/dL/h. Give 10–20 units of regular insulin intravenously immediately, followed by an infusion of 5–10 units per h. Change to a sliding scale when the blood glucose falls below 180 mg/dL.

Treatment of acidosis
There is no evidence that sodium bicarbonate is beneficial and it should not be used routinely.

General measures
Blood, urine, and sputum cultures can be obtained to determine the presence of a suspected infection, in which case broad-spectrum antibiotics can be used in treatment. Deep vein thrombosis (DVT) prophylaxis can also be used. Intubation and ventilation are necessary if the patient is unconscious, or in the event of respiratory failure, which may be suggested by a normal partial pressure of carbon dioxide ($PaCO_2$) in the face of a profound metabolic acidosis; hyperventilate to maintain respiratory compensation. One must assume that the patient has a full stomach, so rapid sequence intubation is required.

Complications
Mortality attributable to DKA is rare when appropriate treatment is given. However, cerebral edema may occur due to excessive fluids or a too rapid correction of hypernatremia. There is also the possibility of DVT, hypoglycemia, and sepsis.

Hyperosmolar nonketotic coma
A hyperosmola nonketotic coma usually occurs in elderly people, in cases where there has been no history of type 1 diabetes, and also where there has been an insidious onset over the preceding weeks.

Clinical features
The clinical features include the following:
- Dehydration – this is the major problem, usually more severe than in DKA, with a fluid deficit of up to 25% of total body water; plasma Na^+ may exceed 155 mmol/L, contributing to hyperosmolality (which may be in excess of 400 mosmol/L).
- Coma, with or without focal neurologic signs.
- Gross hyperglycemia and hyperosmolality – the blood glucose may be greater than 1,000 mg/dL.
- Absence of acidosis/hyperventilation.

Management

General principles are the same as for the management of DKA. If Na^+ exceeds 155 mmol/L, replace fluid losses with 0.45% NaCl. Aim to replace half the estimated deficit within 12 h, and the remainder over the following 24 h. Rapid reductions in plasma osmolality may lead to cerebral edema. Potassium requirements may be high. There is also a high risk of thromboembolism.

Intensive insulin therapy

Normalization of glucose levels (80–110 mg/dL) has been shown to improve survival in one large study of surgical patients. A similar study evaluating medical ICU patients did not demonstrate a survival benefit. This strategy typically involves administration of an insulin infusion and frequent (eg, every 1–2 h) assays of glucose levels. The most common complication with this strategy is hypoglycemia, which must be anticipated and monitored carefully.

Thyroid disorders

The thyroid gland produces triiodothyronine (T_3) and thyroxine (T_4) in response to thyroid-stimulating hormone (TSH). T_3 is biologically active and its actions include:

- heat production (partly due to stimulation of Na^+/K^+ ATPase)
- increased metabolic rate of many tissues
- control of growth and development
- regulation of carbohydrate and fat metabolism.

Myxedema coma

This is a rare condition with high mortality; there is usually long-standing unrecognized hypothyroidism. Precipitating factors include cold weather, intercurrent illness, drugs (particularly central nervous system [CNS] depressants such as general anesthetic agents), and surgery. It is most common in elderly women, and results from either primary thyroid disease or pituitary failure.

Clinical features

The clinical features of a myxedema coma are as follows:

- pre-coma features, such as fatigue, mental dulling/psychosis/depression, cold intolerance, dry skin, hoarseness, constipation, and weight gain
- coma seizures, which complicate the coma in 25% of cases
- hypothermia

- hypotension and bradycardia – EKG changes include low voltage, prolongation of QT interval and flattening/inversion of T-wave, heart failure, and pericardial effusion
- respiratory failure with respiratory acidosis and hypoxia
- metabolic derangements, such as hyponatremia, increased total body water, and reduced plasma osmolality, lactic acidosis, and hypoglycemia
- adrenocortical insufficiency (either as a result of panhypopituitarism or associated autoimmune disease)
- gastrointestinal ileus
- myopathy.

Diagnosis

There is a high index of suspicion in patients presenting with coma and hypothermia. Thyroid function tests (Figure 7.3) can also be carried out. Additional tests that can be performed are pituitary and adrenocortical function tests, including a random cortisol, adrenocorticotropic hormone (ACTH) stimulation, and prolactin test.

Management

Thyroid replacement therapy

There is no accepted regimen for thyroid replacement therapy; specifically, there is debate concerning a number of factors, which are listed below:

- Dose – some advocate large loading dose regimens in view of uncertain enteral absorption, high-capacity protein binding and reduced T_4 to T_3 conversion. Cardiac side effects (arrhythmias, ischemia, sudden death) are more common with higher doses.
- T_4 versus T_3 – 20 mg T_3 is equivalent to 100 mg T_4. The effects of T_4 are smoother but it may take more than 24 h for any response in body temperature, heart rate, or mental state. Response to T_3 may be seen within 4 h,

Thyroid function tests				
Diagnosis	T_3 level	T_4 level	TSH level	RT_3 level
Primary hypothyroidism	↓ or normal	↓	↑ or normal	↑ or normal
Central hypothyroidism	↓	↓	Normal or ↓	↓
Euthyroid sick	↓	↓ or normal	Normal or ↓	↑ or normal

Figure 7.3 Thyroid function tests. RT_3, reverse triiodothyronine; T_3, triiodothyronine; T_4, thyroxine; TSH, thyroid-stimulating hormone.

although cardiac side effects are more common. It is recommended that T_3 be avoided in patients with cardiac disease.

- Route of administration – either agent can be given enterally (although this route may be ineffective because of gastrointestinal ileus and delayed gastric emptying) or parenterally (by either slow bolus injection or continuous infusion).
- Suggested regimens – T_4 300–500 mg IV bolus, followed by 50–100 mg i.v. daily, converted to oral/nasogastric when intestinal function returns; T_3 25–50 mg IV bolus followed by 10–20 mg i.v. 8-hourly, converted to oral/nasogastric T_4 when gastric function returns.
- Assume adrenocortical insufficency and give hydrocortisone 50 mg i.v. 6-hourly.

Hypothermia

Active rewarming is contraindicated as the resulting peripheral vasodilation may provoke hemodynamic collapse.

Cardiorespiratory support

Intubation and ventilation are often required due to coma, hypercapnia, hypoxia, etc. The low metabolic rate means that minute ventilation requirements are low. There is often marked resistance to pressor agents. Beware tracheal compression from goiter.

Hypoglycemia

A dose of 25 g dextrose should be given immediately, followed by an infusion as indicated.

Hyponatremia

Hyponatremia is believed to be due to water retention and inappropriate secretion of antidiuretic hormone (ADH). Fluid restriction is the basis of treatment; hypertonic saline may be considered if Na^+ is less than 120 mmol/L, but beware fluid overload and heart failure.

Thyrotoxic crisis

Thyrotoxic crisis is an extreme and exaggerated variant of hyperthyroidism. It is more common in women, and carries a high mortality.

Causes

Most patients have poorly controlled Graves' disease, the crisis being precipitated by factors such as an infection, trauma, surgery, or DKA.

Other causes include iodine-131 (^{131}I) therapy in previously untreated patients, thyroid surgery in poorly prepared patients, and an overdose of T_4.

Clinical features

The patient may present with a combination of features which may vary – these features are listed below:

- cardiovascular – severe tachyarrhythmias, hyperdynamic circulation, heart failure, increased voltage, and left ventricular hypertrophy on EKG
- respiratory – hyperventilation to deal with increased CO_2 production, breathlessness
- hyperpyrexia – may be >40°C
- neurologic – anxiety, tremor, weakness, confusion, coma
- gastrointestinal – diarrhea, nausea and vomiting, abdominal pain, weight loss, hepatic failure
- metabolic – dehydration, hyponatremia, hypokalemia
- goiter.

Management

β Blockade addresses the hyperadrenergic state and inhibits peripheral conversion of T_4 to T_3. Propranolol can be administered in incremental 0.5 mg IV boluses to maximum of 5 mg, maintenance 40–160 mg 6-hourly orally. Asthma, heart failure, and heart block are relative contraindications. Esmolol is a useful alternative to propranolol, and can be given by continuous IV infusion: 500 mg/kg over 2 min followed by infusion of 50–200 mg/kg per min.

Antithyroid treatment can be methimazole, a 25 mg dose administered every 6 h, or propylthiouracil 200–250 mg every 6 h, orally, or via nasogastric tube. Iodine inhibits the synthesis and release of thyroid hormones. Do not give for at least 1 h after methimazole/propylthiouracil. Give as saturated solution potassium iodide (ssKI) one drop (50 mg) every 12 h. Lithium carbonate is useful in patients allergic to iodine, 500–1,500 mg daily, therapeutic range 0.7–1.4 mmol/L.

Antiarrhythmics such as digoxin can be administered in large doses if required; however, it is important to be aware of hypokalemia. Amiodarone has the additional benefit of inhibiting T_4 to T_3 conversion.

Corticosteroids (eg, intravenous hydrocortisone) can be administered in doses of 50–100 mg every 6 h.

Metabolic management involves administering IV fluids to combat dehydration; use central venous pressure (CVP)/pulmonary capillary wedge pressure (PCWP) monitoring in heart failure. Nutritional requirements are high, so commence feeding early (attempt enteral feeding first, resort to parenteral route if not tolerated). Maintain a high normal K^+ in view of risk of arrhythmias.

Subcutaneous heparin is associated with a high risk of DVT.

Other measures such as a fan or tepid sponging can help to control pyrexia; aspirin displaces thyroid hormones from binding proteins and is contraindicated. Intubation, mechanical ventilation, and occasionally neuromuscular blockade may be necessary to help control hypermetabolism. Plasmapheresis may be of benefit in refractory cases.

Adrenocortical and pituitary insufficiency

Adrenocortical insufficiency

The adrenal cortex produces three classes of steroid hormone: sex hormones, glucocorticoids (cortisol), and mineralocorticoids (aldosterone). The normal daily production of cortisol is 30 mg/day, which can increase to up to 300 mg/day under severe stress. Cortisol has a permissive action on carbohydrate, fat, and protein metabolism, and also has CNS, renal, and immunomodulatory effects. It maintains vascular responsiveness. The stress response is essential for survival.

Production is regulated by ACTH secreted by the pituitary gland. Aldosterone is responsible for the defense of Na^+ and extracellular fluid volume. Its secretion is controlled by the renin/angiotensin system and extracellular K^+. It is not dependent on ACTH.

Causes

One cause is primary Addison's disease (which results in sepsis), autoimmune disease, infection (eg, tuberculosis, meningococci, fungi), neoplastic infiltration, hemorrhagic shock, critical illness, and cytotoxic drugs. One study demonstrated a survival benefit in patients with septic shock who received low-dose hydrocortisone (50 mg i.v. every 6 h) and fludrocortisone (50 μg orally every day) for 7 days. The benefit was limited to those who did not respond to ACTH stimulation testing (250 μg ACTH with cortisol measured 30 and 60 min later). Nonresponders were defined as those who did not increase cortisol levels greater than 9 μg/dL.

Secondary ACTH deficiency – pituitary failure and cessation of long-term steroid therapy (which induces adrenal atrophy via suppression of ACTH synthesis).

Clinical features

Clinical features are variable and depend upon the cause and speed of onset. Features of acute decompensation include lethargy, muscle weakness, weight loss, confusion, abdominal pain, hypotension and cardiovascular collapse, hyponatremia, hyperkalemia, and hypoglycemia. There may be coexisting endocrine abnormalities. Pigmentation is a feature of chronic primary disease, and is a result of the increased secretion of the ACTH precursor pro-opiomelanocortin. Secondary hypoadrenalism tends to be less severe because aldosterone secretion is preserved. An acute addisonian crisis may go unrecognized in critically ill patients, in whom the clinical features are nonspecific. It should be considered in any patient with unexplained hypotension, particularly if associated with characteristic biochemical disturbances (hyperkalemia, hyponatremia, hypoglycemia).

Diagnosis
The following list can be used as a guide to aid diagnosis:
- clinical suspicion
- biochemical features
- low random cortisol
- loss of cortisol response to ACTH (ACTH stimulation test)
- adrenal antibodies, abdominal X-ray (adrenal calcification), and adrenal and pituitary CT.

Management
Cardiovascular support involves using 0.9% NaCl to resuscitate the extracellular fluid (ECF) deficit; large volumes may be required, and should be guided by measurement of CVP and hourly urine output. Vasopressors may be necessary in severe cases; high doses may be required.

Steroid therapy involves hydrocortisone 50 mg i.v. every 6 h, and mineralocorticoid (fludrocortisone 50–100 μg orally daily).

A 50% solution of dextrose can be given, as necessary, to treat hypoglycemia. Management of adrenocortical insufficiency also involves treating the precipitating cause – an addisonian crisis will usually develop only when the stress response fails to develop in response to an appropriate stimulus.

Panhypopituitarism
The anterior lobe of the pituitary gland controls the release of thyroid, adrenocortical, and gonadal sex hormones, and directly synthesizes growth hormone. The posterior lobe releases ADH and oxytocin.

Causes
The causes of panhypopituitarism include:
- neoplasm (eg, adenomas, craniopharyngioma, metastasis)
- ischemia

- infection/inflammation (eg, tuberculosis, meningitis, sarcoid)
- physical injury (eg, surgery, radiotherapy, trauma).

Clinical features

The clinical features of presentation of pituitary insufficiency depend on the cause and its time course. For instance, a pituitary macroadenoma secreting growth hormone that has destroyed the rest of the anterior lobe will present with a combination of the features of excess growth hormone (acromegaly or gigantism) along with those of thyroid, adrenocortical, and gonadal insufficiency. It is less common for the posterior lobe to be involved, although diabetes insipidus (DI) may develop.

Diagnosis

This depends on a high index of suspicion, and treatment cannot wait for laboratory confirmation. Blood should be sent for random cortisol, thyroid function, prolactin, and growth hormone assays. A CT scan of the head should be carried out when the condition of the patient allows; this may confirm the diagnosis of a pituitary tumor or infarction and will exclude any associated hydrocephalus that might require urgent drainage. Dynamic tests of pituitary function (eg, glucagon stimulation test) should be performed at a later date under the guidance of an endocrinologist experienced in pituitary disorders.

Treatment

Adrenocortical and thyroid insufficiency should be treated as described elsewhere, as should DI. Patients with gross acromegaly present particular problems that require specific treatment. Problems include hypertrophy of the soft tissues of the airway leading to obstructive sleep apnea, difficulties with airway maintenance under anesthesia, and difficult intubation. Hypertension and cardiomyopathy, and glucose intolerance may also occur. Figure 7.4 provides a dosage guide to using steroids.

Hypocalcemia

Causes

The causes of hypocalcemia include:
- hypoparathyroidism – surgery, severe sepsis
- vitamin D deficiency – decreased gastrointestinal absorption, renal failure, liver disease
- calcium-losing states – increased uptake into bone ('hungry bones'), pancreatitis, rhabdomyolysis, hyperphosphataemia (by causing ectopic calcifi-

Equivalent steroid dosages

Agent	Equivalent anti-inflammatory dose (mg)	Mineralocorticoid activity
Hydrocortisone (cortisol)	20	++
Cortisone	25	++
Prednisolone	5	+
Prednisone	5	+
Dexamethasone	0.75	0
Betamethasone	0.75	0
Methylprednisolone	4	0
Triamcinolone	4	0

Figure 7.4 Equivalent steroid dosages.

cation), chelating agents (ethylenediaminetetraacetic acid [EDTA], citrate, radiographic contrast media)

- calcium shifts – alkalosis (decreases ionized Ca^{2+}), free fatty acids (increase Ca^{2+} binding to albumin).

Clinical features

Clinical features result from a fall in the ionized Ca^{2+}, and are more severe when the fall is rapid rather than gradual. They can be grouped accordingly:

- neuromuscular – weakness, hyperreflexia, tetany, muscle spasms/cramps, seizures, positive Trousseau's sign (paresthesia and carpopedal spasm following inflation of BP cuff > systolic pressure for 3 min)
- psychiatric – anxiety, confusion, psychosis, depression, lethargy
- cardiovascular – hypotension, heart failure, heart block, ventricular fibrillation, resistance to digoxin, catecholamines, prolonged QT, ST intervals, T-wave inversion.

Investigations

Investigations that can be carried out include ionized Ca^{2+}, parathyroid hormone (PTH) assay, serum phosphate (PO_4^{3-}), serum magnesium (Mg^{2+}) as hypomagnesemia contributes to consequences of hypocalcemia, and renal function.

Treatment

Treament is generally not indicated for asymptomatic hypocalcemia. General supportive measures can be adopted: calcium supplements administered intravenously in 10 mL 10% calcium gluconate over 5–10 minutes, followed by an infusion of 2–10 mL/h, while checking ionized Ca^{2+} regularly; 10 mL 10%

calcium gluconate is equivalent to 2.25 mmol Ca^{2+} (10 mL 10% calcium chloride is equivalent to 6.8 mmol Ca^{2+}). Correct hypomagnesemia as deficits may be 0.5–1 mmol/kg, and up to 2 mmol/kg replacement may be necessary to account for urinary losses, given over 5 days. Give 1–2 g magnesium sulfate as a slow bolus followed by continuous IV infusion of 2–8 g/day. Use lower dose in renal failure. Oral administration is usually ineffective. Treat vitamin D deficiency (0.25 mg calcitriol daily orally).

Hypercalcemia

Total plasma Ca^{2+} = 8.8–10 mmol/L, of which 40% is bound to plasma proteins, 10% chelated, and 50% the free ionized form. The last is immediately biologically active. Plasma Ca^{2+} is influenced by a number of factors, as shown in the figure on the next page. Severe hypercalcemia (total Ca^{2+} >12 mg/dL) can be life threatening. Acute shifts in Ca^{2+} from bone to extracellular fluid (ECF) are the most important causes of hypercalcemia. A prominent feature is the depletion of the ECF compartment due to impairment of the ability of the kidney to retain Na^+/water. This causes renal hypoperfusion and further impairs the ability of the kidneys to excrete Ca^{2+}.

Causes

These are primary hyperparathyroidism, from a parathyroid adenoma or ectopic source (bronchogenic carcinoma, hypernephroma), and metastatic malignancy, multiple myeloma, excess Ca^{2+}/vitamin D intake, sarcoidosis, and Paget's disease.

Clinical features

Dehydration, cardiovascular collapse, prolonged QT interval on EKG, general malaise, and muscle weakness are all notable features. Other clinical signs include altered conscious levels, anorexia, nausea and vomiting, constipation, abdominal pain, renal colic, and ectopic calcification (conjunctivitis, pruritis).

Investigations

Ionized Ca^{2+} is preferable to total calcium, which is influenced by changes in the concentration of plasma-binding proteins. It should ideally be a sample taken without the use of a tourniquet (because increases in venous pressure may influence the concentration of plasma proteins). Many blood gas analyzers now have a Ca^{2+}-selective electrode.

It is also important to search for the cause; PTH assay, parathyroid imaging, chest X-ray (eg, bronchogenic carcinoma, metastatic disease), bone scan, skull

X-ray (eg, multiple myeloma), and kidney and upper bladder X-ray (eg, renal tract stones) can all be used to determine the presence of hypercalcemia. Complete blood count, renal function, phosphate, alkaline phosphatase, plasma, and urine electrophoresis can also be carried out.

Management
If the patient is severely hypotensive or unconscious, admit to the ICU, with arterial and CVP lines and continuous EKG and SaO_2 monitoring. Rehydrate with 0.9% NaCl. Specific calcium-lowering therapies include the following:

- Calciuresis: forced diuresis with 0.9% NaCl and furosemide 5–10 mg/h. Only start when adequate rehydration has been achieved; hypovolemia, hypokalemia, and hypomagnesemia are potential risks.
- Inhibitors of bone resorption.
- Bisphosphonates: eg, pamidronate 15–60 mg as slow infusion or in divided doses over 2–4 days; maximum of 90 mg per treatment course.
- Mithramycin: 25 mg/kg i.v. as bolus or infusion. Effective for up to 6 days. Risk of thrombocytopenia and hepatic impairment when repeated doses are given.
- Calcitonin: 3–4 IU/kg i.v. initially, followed by up to 8 IU subcutaneously 6- to 12-hourly. Tachyphylaxis often develops within several days.
- Steroids: hydrocortisone 50–100 mg i.v. 6-hourly or prednisone 10–25 mg/day. Act by inhibiting gastrointestinal absorption and bone resorption. Useful in hypercalcemia associated with malignancy. Effect takes some days to develop.
- Treatment of cause: eg, parathyroidectomy, tumor irradiation.

Treat hypokalemia as appropriate; exhibit caution in treating hypophosphatemia since ectopic calcification becomes more likely when the Ca^{2+}/PO_4^{3-} solubility product exceeds 75.

Chapter 8

Gastrointestinal disorders

Imre Noth
University of Chicago, Chicago, IL, USA

Gastrointestinal integrity in critically ill individuals

Background

Within 24 h of admission the majority of critically ill patients will develop stress-related mucosal damage. Clinically relevant bleeding causes hematemesis and/or melena; hypotension, tachycardia, or anemia occurs in 1–4% of patients. Those who develop stress-related mucosal disease, endoscopic signs of bleeding, or clinically important bleeding have a higher risk of death.

Mechanisms

Compromise of the mucosal lining may be the result of splanchnic ischemia and has two principal consequences – acid pepsin attacks and bacterial translocation.

Acid pepsin attacks the mucosa of the upper gastrointestinal (GI) tract, leading to peptic erosions or ulcerations and the risk of hemorrhage. Bacterial translocation is the passage of gut bacteria or their toxins across a disrupted intestinal mucosa into the portal circulation and therefore systemically. It is believed that such leakage fuels the inflammatory processes of systemic inflammation and multiple organ dysfunction syndrome (*see* Chapter 9).

Major factors that contribute to splanchnic ischemia and consequently stress ulcer formation are a decreased blood flow, mucosal ischemia, hypoperfusion, and reperfusion injury. Mucosal integrity depends on an intact microcirculation. The mucous layer that protects the surface of the epithelium from hydrogen ions may be compromised when hypoperfusion and acidosis combine to decrease gastric blood flow. This may be a major factor in stress-related mucosal bleeding.

Causes

Etiologies believed to lead to a breakdown of these defenses are:

- respiratory failure
- coagulopathy
- hypotension
- sepsis
- hepatic failure
- renal failure
- glucocorticoids.

Acid production and suppression

Gastric acid release is stimulated by food. When a meal containing protein is consumed, amino acids are released, stimulating the release of gastrin by G cells in the antrum. This, in turn, stimulates the enterochromaffin-like (ECL) cells of the stomach to release histamine. Nocturnal histamine release may be regulated by a pituitary adenylyl cyclase-activating polypeptide that is neurally released.

Parietal cells, located in the body and fundus of the stomach, are involved in the production of gastric acid. In response to various stimuli, these cells secrete hydrogen ions. Nearby ECL cells, stimulated by gastrin, then secrete histamine which binds to specific receptors on the parietal cells. Calcium may also play a role by stimulating parietal cells to release acid or by causing G cells to stimulate the release of gastrin. Acid suppression may therefore be achieved by various means:

- direct acid neutralization, such as antacids
- blockade of stimulation of parietal cell along the cascade by histamine and gastrin
- blockade of cholinergic pathways
- blockade of the acid-producing proton pump at the parietal cell.

Management in the intensive care setting

Acid suppression

There are several therapies available for ensuring GI integrity in the critically ill patient in the intensive care unit (ICU) as shown in Figure 8.1. Proton-pump inhibitors (PPIs) are the first agent of choice. There are two major forms for acid suppression: H_2-receptor blockers and PPIs.

H_2-receptor blockers (eg, ranitidine) block those pathways mediated by histamine. They cannot, however, block sites mediated by other pathways, specifically gastrin and acetylcholine receptor pathways. While they may

Commonly used gastric acid-related drugs

Drugs	Dosage
H$_2$-receptor blockers	
Cimetidine	300 mg i.v./i.m./p.o. q 6–8 h
Famotidine	20 mg i.v., 20–40 mg p.o. twice daily
Nizatidine	150–300 mg p.o. twice daily
Ranitidine	150 mg p.o. bid, 50 mg i.v./i.m. q 8 h
Proton-pump inhibitors	
Esomeprazole	20–40 mg p.o. q day. Also available as an IV preparation
Lansoprazole	15–30 mg p.o. q day. Also available as an IV preparation
Omeprazole	20–40 mg p.o. q day
Pantoprazole	10–40 mg p.o. q day. Also available as an IV preparation
Rabeprazole	10–20 mg p.o. q day
Synthetic prostaglandin E$_1$ analog	
Misoprostol	100 mg p.o. b.i.d.
Other	
Sucralfate	1–2 g p.o. qAC and qHS

Figure 8.1 Commonly used gastric acid-related drugs. IV, intravenous; qAC, dose to be taken before meals; qHS, dose to be taken once a day at bedtime.

reduce the risk of stress-related mucosal disease, they do not treat clinically important bleeding from a peptic ulcer. H$_2$-receptor antagonists are able to elevate pH levels only above 4.0. This level of acid suppression appears to be insufficient to control or prevent rebleeding episodes. In addition, tachyphylaxis appears to develop to continuous IV infusion within 72 h.

PPIs block histamine H$_2$-receptors, gastrin, and cholinergically mediated sources. These class of drugs are weak bases that when activated bind to the proton pump and inhibit its ability to produce gastric acid. For intravenous use, omeprazole, esomeprazole, and pantoprazole are available. The ease of use, reliability of elevation of gastric pH, and absence of clinically significant drug interactions make pantoprazole an attractive therapy in emergency settings, such as acute upper GI hemorrhage, high-risk stress ulcer patients, and patients who cannot tolerate an oral PPI.

There are several advantages of using PPIs, such as pantoprazole, in the ICU setting. Maintenance of an elevated intragastric pH has the potential to prevent stress-related mucosal disease. Studies have demonstrated that a pH of more than 4.0 is adequate to prevent stress ulceration. However, a pH greater than

6.0 may be necessary to maintain clotting in patients at risk from rebleeding in peptic ulcer disease. Preliminary data suggest that intravenous doses of a PPI (eg, pantoprazole) administered intermittently to critically ill patients, who could not receive enteral feeding, are as effective in raising intragastric pH to more than 4.0 on the first day as continuous high-dose infusions of intravenous H_2-receptor antagonists. Pantoprazole has been demonstrated to increase gastric pH to more than 6.0 in a bolus dose of 80 mg followed with continuous infusion of 8 mg/h. In trials in the ICU setting, this level of suppression demonstrates a significant reduction in rebleeding and the need for surgery. Specifically, intravenous pantoprazole, at the above-mentioned dose, more reliably maintained that level of acid suppression than intravenous famotidine. Furthermore, the oral preparation of pantoprazole appears to carry the same level of suppression.

There are, however, concerns that the elevation in pH in patients may lead to increased episodes of pneumonia. Drug interactions occur as PPIs are metabolized by the cytochrome P450 system. Omeprazole has the highest potential for drug interactions because it inhibits several cytochrome enzymes. Current common usage practices in emergency settings in countries where pantoprazole has been available are: initiation with a bolus of 80 mg i.v. followed by continuous infusion for 72 h with change to oral dosing at that time.

It is also important to ensure that there is adequate oxygenation of the splanchnic area.

Sucralfate

A dosage of sucralfate 1–2 g nasogastrically every 4–6 h is also recommended. A complex of aluminium hydroxide and sulfated sucrose is thought to act by protecting the gastric mucosa from an acid pepsin attack. It requires an acid environment to act, and should not therefore be combined with H_2-receptor blockade or PPIs. It should be used with caution in renal failure (accumulation of aluminum). Gastric acidity is maintained, which may also help to protect against nosocomial pneumonia.

Enteral nutrition

Enteral nutrition combats stress ulceration and helps maintain intestinal mucosal integrity. A daily rest period allows gastric acidity to be restored, and many believe that patients on full enteral feeding regimens require no other prophylaxis.

Other measures include antacids, and prostaglandin E_1 analogs although, in general, these are less effective than the therapies discussed above.

Choosing whom to treat

Not all patients have the same risk of developing clinically significant, stress-related mucosal disease and stress-related upper GI bleeding. In the setting of the ICU two groups of patients warrant acid suppression: those with a high risk of GI bleeding, and patients with upper GI bleeding. Those with a high risk of GI bleeding (eg, stress ulcers), and who should therefore receive prophylaxis, include:

- those who require mechanical ventilation for more than 48 h
- patients with a coagulopathy
- patients in hypotensive shock
- patients with burns
- patients with a history of peptic ulcer disease.

Risk was increased 16-fold in the mechanical ventilation group and fourfold in the coagulopathy group. Patients with upper gastrointestinal bleeding should receive acid suppression as prophylaxis, because it also prevents rebleeding.

Gastric tonometry

The adequacy of splanchnic perfusion can be estimated from gastric intramucosal pH (pH_i), which is, in turn, derived from measurement of the arterial hydrogen carbonate (HCO_3^-) concentration and gut mucosal partial pressure of carbon dioxide ($PaCO_2$). The latter is measured using a gastric tonometer as illustrated in Figure 8.2. Once positioned, the silicone balloon of the tonometer is filled with 2.5 mL 0.9% saline and, after allowing sufficient time for equilibration of CO_2 between the mucosa and the balloon (30 min or more), anaerobic samples of tonometer saline and arterial blood are taken simultaneously and blood gas analysis performed. The steady-state $PaCO_2$ ($PaCO_{2[ss]}$) is obtained from the measured $PaCO_2$ adjusted for the time taken for equilibration using a slide calculator provided with the kit. The pH_i is obtained from the Henderson–Hasselbalch equation:

$$pH_i = 6.1 + \log_{10}\{[HCO_3^-]_{art}/(PaCO_{2[ss]}) \times 0.031\}$$

Various assumptions are made:

- Mucosal $PaCO_2$ is in equilibrium with that of the luminal contents and the saline-filled balloon.
- The tissue HCO_3^- concentration is the same as that of arterial blood.
- Plasma and tissue pK_a values are the same.

Measurement of pH_i is unaffected by concomitant administration of H_2-receptor antagonists or sucralfate. The normal value for pH_i is greater than 7.35.

Gastric tonometry

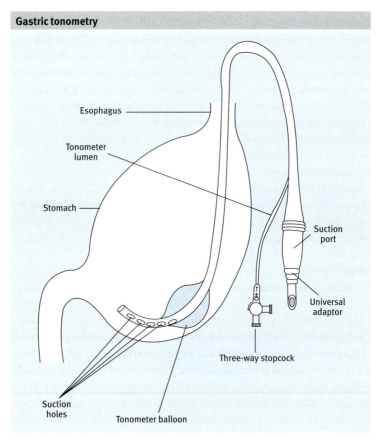

Figure 8.2 Gastric tonometry.

Bleeding esophageal varices

Esophageal varices are collateral channels between the portal and systemic venous circulations (left gastric to esophageal), which develop as a result of portal hypertension (ie, >20 mmHg, normal 5–10 mmHg).

Management

Patients with bleeding esophageal varices should be managed in an ICU.

Resuscitation

It is important to check full blood count and hematocrit, urea and electrolytes, blood glucose, and clotting factors such as prothrombin, thromboplastin, international normalized ratio (INR), and platelets. Follow this by cross-matching 2–8 units of blood immediately and request 15 mL/kg fresh frozen plasma (FFP). If feasible, insert two large-bore (18 gauge or better) peripheral intravenous cannulae, and a central venous pressure (CVP) line, but not at the expense of delaying resuscitation. Transfuse with colloid, blood, and clotting factors (including calcium and platelets) according to clinical measures of resuscitation (urine output, peripheral perfusion, heart rate, blood pressure). It is best to avoid 0.9% saline because this may precipitate ascites.

Management of encephalopathy

The altered conscious level associated with fulminant hepatic failure may be precipitated by infection, drugs, or GI hemorrhage (high protein load) (see also section on acute liver failure). Treatment includes:

- identification and treatment of cause
- enemas and lactulose to empty the bowel
- enteral neomycin to sterilize bowel contents
- measurement and treatment of raised intracranial pressure.

Vasoactive drugs

Vasopressin (0.3–0.6 units/min) causes generalized vasoconstriction and controls bleeding in approximately 50–60% of cases. However, there is a risk of ischemia of other organs and, therefore, nitroglycerin is often used simultaneously. Rebleeding is also common. Somatostatin (and the synthetic analog octreotide) controls bleeding from varices by reducing flow in splanchnic vessels and reducing portal venous pressure. Gastric acid secretion is also reduced.

Endoscopic sclerotherapy

Sclerotherapy controls bleeding in approximately 70–80% of cases. Similar success is achieved with banding of various lesions. Banding may have advantages of more rapid ablation and fewer episodes of recurrence. General anesthesia may be required. Possible complications include perforation, ulcers, and stricture formation. Sclerotherapy can be repeated if the patient rebleeds.

Balloon tamponade

Balloon tamponade controls bleeding in 70–80% of cases, but rebleeding is common. The Minnesota modification of the Sengstaken–Blakemore tube should be used; there are four channels:

1. Gastric lumen.
2. Esophageal lumen.

3. Gastric balloon.
4. Esophageal balloon.

To insert, place the patient in a head-down lateral position, pass the tube to the 50 cm mark, and confirm this position in the stomach. Empty the stomach by aspiration, inflate the gastric balloon with 200–350 mL air, saline, or contrast, and apply firm traction (1–2 kg applied to tube via pulley and cord). The esophageal balloon should be inflated to 35–40 mmHg if the gastric balloon fails to control bleeding, but should not be inflated for more than 24 h. Complications include esophageal necrosis, rupture, and aspiration pneumonia.

Portosystemic shunting
Portosystemic shunting should be used if patients continue to bleed despite conservative treatment. Anastomosis of the portal and systemic circulations reduces portal pressure and hence reduces bleeding from varices. Transjugular intrahepatic portosystemic shunt (TIPS) is the procedure of choice as it is associated with a lower morbidity and mortality compared with surgical shunting. A catheter is passed into the hepatic vein via the internal jugular vein and a metal stent inserted. Surgical shunts should be performed on patients in whom TIPS has failed or is contraindicated (eg, right heart failure, portal vein thrombosis). Portosystemic shunts may precipitate encephalopathy. The risk of encephalopathy is reduced if a selective decompression is performed (eg, distal splenorenal shunt), compared with a portocaval anastomosis that decompresses the entire splanchnic bed.

Esophageal transection
Esophageal transection can be performed if TIPS fails or is not available. The feeding vessels are ligated and the esophagus reanastomosed.

Liver transplantation
Liver transplantation should be considered in cases of recurrent bleeding despite the above measures.

Zollinger–Ellison syndrome
Definition
Hypergastrinemia from a gastrinoma tumor causes Zollinger–Ellison syndrome (ZES) leading to gastric acid hypersecretion. Gastrin leads to hypertrophy and hyperplasia of the parietal cells which, in turn, also results in gastric acid hypersecretion. Although a rare disease, it is life threatening. It can lead to severe reflux or peptic ulcer disease that is often refractory and severe.

Diagnosis

The diagnosis should be considered in patients with duodenal ulcer and diarrhea, peptic ulcers in unusual locations, or multiple ulcers refractory to treatment. Diagnosis requires elevation of fasting hypergastrinemia leading to an increased basal gastric acid output. PPIs should be discontinued for 1 week prior to diagnosis.

Management

The control of gastric acid secretion represents a significant challenge. The objective of gastric acid control in ZES is to reduce the acid output to normal ranges. Oral PPIs are effective in achieving control. Pantoprazole administered intravenously can attain normal acid secretion levels at a dose of 80 mg twice daily and is approved by the Food and Drug Administration for this indication. Patients can be switched from oral to intravenous (IV) in the event of hospitalization, critical illness, or during the perioperative period for surgical resection.

ZES can be cured in 30% of patients by surgical resection. More than 50% of patients with control of acid hypersecretion who are not cured will die of tumor-related causes. Surgical resection should, therefore, be pursued whenever possible.

Acute liver failure

Definition

There should be no history or evidence of pre-existing liver disease:

- hyperacute (7 days)
- acute (8–28 days)
- subacute (5–12 weeks).

Patients with a faster onset of encephalopathy tend to have a better prognosis.

Causes

Acute liver failure can be cause by several factors, such as:

- acetaminophen overdose (eg, 50% of cases in the UK)
- viral hepatitis (eg, 40% of cases in the UK and 70% outside the UK) – hepatitis A, B, C, D, and E, herpes simplex virus I and II, herpes zoster virus, cytomegalovirus, Epstein–Barr virus
- other drugs – halothane, ethanol, isoniazid, rifampin, nonsteroidal anti-inflammatory drugs, monoamine oxidase inhibitors, sodium valproate, methyldopa

- fatty liver of pregnancy
- Wilson's disease
- Reye's syndrome
- hyperthermia syndromes
- massive malignant infiltration
- galactosemia
- amyloid.

Presentation

One of the clearest signs of acute liver failure is jaundice. Other signs include: hepatic fetor, asterixis (ie, flapping tremor), encephalopathy (ie, confusion and obtundation), hepatomegaly, and spider nevi, which are a sign of chronic disease but can occur in severe acute disease. Deranged liver function tests are also necessary and may reveal massively elevated levels of aminotransferase (although low levels may eventually follow when hepatocyte destruction is complete). Elevated levels of phosphatase, bilirubin, and prothrombin time (PT)/INR (ie, clotting failure) may also be detected by liver function tests.

Principles of management

Successful management of acute liver failure involves identifying the cause and removing it where possible, as in the case of charcoal hemoperfusion. Further hepatocyte damage can be prevented by optimizing oxygenation and perfusion. It is also important to look for possible complications and treat them accordingly. Regeneration of hepatocytes can be promoted using drugs such as insulin, glucagon, norepinephrine, vasopressin, angiotensin, estrogens, and hepatocyte growth factor. At present, the mainstay of treatment is preservation of remaining function rather than hepatocyte regeneration. Early recognition of the patient who may require a liver transplantation is essential.

Indications for liver transplantation

There are several indications for liver transplantation. The guidelines used at King's College Hospital, London in the UK, are as follows:

- acetaminophen induced – pH <7.3, or partial thromboplastin time (PTT) >100 seconds and creatinine >300 mmol/L and grade III/IV encephalopathy
- non-acetaminophen induced – PTT >100 seconds, or any three of the following:
  - age <10 years or >40 years

- etiology: non-A, non-B viral hepatitis, halothane hepatitis, drug reaction
- jaundice has duration of >7 days before onset of encephalopathy
- PTT >50 seconds
- serum bilirubin >300 mmol/L.

Complications of acute liver failure
Encephalopathy

This is a fluctuating mental state progressing to coma, associated with increased activity of the inhibitory neurotransmitter γ-aminobutyric acid. Contributing or precipitating/exacerbating factors include infection, high protein load in the gut (including GI hemorrhage), electrolyte disturbance, hypoglycemia, and sedative drugs.

As a coma develops, intubation may be necessary to control and protect the airway. Early intervention to secure the airway may prevent aspiration. Seizures may occur and must be treated promptly. Figure 8.3 lists the different classifications of encephalopathy.

Cerebral edema and raised intracranial pressure

Raised intracranial pressure (ICP) is associated with grades III and IV encephalopathy. Some advocate ICP monitoring in ventilated patients. Volume resuscitation and vasoconstrictors are implemented to increase mean arterial pressure (MAP). A cerebral perfusion pressure (ie, the difference between MAP and ICP) of 60 mmHg or more should be maintained. Paralysis, adequate sedation, careful positioning, and mannitol are used to reduce ICP. Stimulation of the patient should be kept to a minimum. If muscle relaxants are used, electrical activity of the brain should be monitored using an electroencephalogram or a cerebral function monitor to detect convulsions.

Measures to control elevated ICP include elevation of the head of the bed, hyperventilation to a $PaCO_2$ that is less than 30 mmHg, and mannitol, administered intravenously usually as 0.5 g/kg IV bolus. The patient may sometimes be given IV sodium thiopental or another sedative.

Classification of encephalopathy

Grade I	Fluctuating confusion, disordered sleep, euphoria, slowed thinking
Grade II	Inappropriate behavior and increasing drowsiness
Grade III	Severe confusion, very drowsy but rousable, obeys simple commands
Grade IV	Coma, may respond to painful stimuli

Figure 8.3 Classification of encephalopathy. Grades II–IV are associated with an abnormal electroencephalogram.

Metabolic and electrolyte disturbances

Hypoglycemia occurs as a result of increased insulin levels and a failure of hepatic gluconeogenesis. Blood glucose should be checked hourly and a glucose infusion given if necessary. Hypokalemia occurs due to vomiting and secondary hyperaldosteronism. Other disturbances that may be present include: dilutional hyponatremia, hypernatremia, and hypomagnesemia (usually iatrogenic), hypophosphatemia, and hypocalcemia. Acid–base disturbances may also occur; for example, abnormalities in the central nervous system (CNS) may induce hyperventilation and a respiratory alkalosis. Metabolic acidosis is more common in acetaminophen/paracetamol poisoning and is associated with a poor prognosis. Lactic acidosis develops in the later stages of the disease as a result of poor tissue perfusion and impaired oxygen extraction. Renal failure may also happen.

Renal failure

Renal failure occurs as a result of the hepatorenal syndrome or direct renal toxicity (eg, acetaminophen/paracetamol overdose) and is associated with a worse outcome. Plasma urea is a poor guide of renal function as production will be reduced. Maintain MAP above 70 mmHg with fluid and inotropes. Dopamine infusion may be of benefit. Intermittent hemodialysis may be poorly tolerated, and continuous techniques of renal support are preferred. Renal function returns with a successful liver transplantation.

Hyperdynamic shock (ie, high cardiac output, low systemic vascular resistance) is very common. The use of epinephrine and/or norepinephrine will increase MAP but reduces oxygen uptake.

Respiratory dysfunction

Respiratory dysfunction may result from aspiration pneumonia/pneumonitis, CNS-driven hyperventilation, fluid overload (particularly if associated with acute renal failure), and acute lung injury caused by sepsis or as part of the spectrum of systemic inflammation. Treatment consists of oxygen therapy, intubation, and mechanical ventilation before protective airway reflexes are lost, antibiotics for infection, and physiotherapy. Bronchoscopy, when indicated, should be exercised with caution in patients with raised ICP.

Coagulopathy

Causes include reduced synthesis/release of clotting factors by failing liver, increased consumption, thrombocytopenia, and hypocalcemia. Hemorrhage from the GI tract, nose, puncture sites, etc. is common. Bleeding from the GI tract can be reduced by the prophylactic use of H_2-receptor antagonists. Blood loss should be replaced with whole blood if possible. FFP and cryoprecipitate should be given as necessary, guided by clotting studies. If the platelet count is less than 50×10^9/L, platelets should be administered prior to invasive procedures or if the patient is bleeding. Coagulation must be checked and corrected prior to insertion of an ICP-monitoring device.

Nosocomial infection is also common. Cultures should be taken often and antibiotics used when indicated. The routine use of prophylactic broad-spectrum antibiotics is advocated by some, but may promote opportunistic infections.

Acute severe pancreatitis

Causes
Acute severe pancreatitis can manifest for a number of reasons. Excessive alcohol consumption is a well-known contributing factor. Biliary tract stones, metabolic disorders (eg, hypercalcemia, hyperlipidemia), and trauma are also recognized factors. Other causes include drugs (eg, steroids, oral contraceptive pill, thiazides), obstructive lesions of the biliary tract (eg, tumor, infection – mumps, Coxsackievirus), idiopathic causes, and iatrogenic causes, such as surgery or endoscopic retrograde cholangiopancreatography.

Diagnosis
Symptoms include abdominal pain radiating to the back, nausea, and vomiting. Signs such as tenderness and guarding, ileus, pyrexia, retroperitoneal bleeding leading to bruising around the flanks (ie, Grey Turner's sign) and umbilicus (ie, Cullen's sign) should also be noted. Recommended diagnostic tests include:
- serum amylase (>1200 U suggests diagnosis)
- a baseline complete blood count, urea and electrolytes, blood glucose, calcium, clotting screen, type and cross-match
- a plain abdominal X-ray
- an abdominal ultrasound scan
- a CT scan.

Indications of severe disease
Figure 8.4 shows indications of severe disease. If the patient meets three or more of these criteria severe disease is indicated.

Pathophysiology
Systemic release of pancreatic toxins can lead to systemic inflammatory response syndrome, associated with variable degrees of shock and tissue hypoperfusion. Local spread leads to retroperitoneal hemorrhage, ileus, splanchnic ischemia,

Indications of severe disease	
Age	>55 years
Blood glucose	>10 mmol/L
Blood urea	>16 mmol/L
Serum albumin	<30 g/L
Serum calcium	<2 mmol/L
Serum aminotransferase	>200 U/L
Serum lactate dehydrogenase	>600 U/L
PaO_2	<8 kPa (60 mmHg)
White cell count	$>15 \times 10^9$/L

Figure 8.4 Indications of severe disease. PaO_2, partial pressure of oxygen.

abscess formation, etc. The condition is often complicated by multiple organ dysfunction and carries a mortality rate that is greater than 10%.

Management

Pain relief
Opioids will be required, but avoid morphine in gallstone-related disease as it constricts the sphincter of Oddi.

Fluid replacement and cardiovascular support
Fluid requirements may be high due to systemic vasodilation, pyrexia, and third-space losses. Therapy should be guided by clinical measures such as urine output, peripheral perfusion, along with CVP monitoring. A pulmonary artery flotation catheter (PAFC) may be required in severe cases. Along with aggressive fluid therapy, inotropes and vasopressors may be required to preserve organ perfusion. Maintain MAP above 70 mmHg.

Correction of electrolyte and acid–base abnormalities
These include hypocalcemia, hypomagnesemia, hypoalbuminemia, and metabolic acidosis (which may be secondary to impaired tissue perfusion).

Nasogastric suction
This is used to reduce vomiting, abdominal distension, and delivery of gastric contents to the duodenum.

Antacid therapy
Ranitidine (50 mg i.v. three times a day, but reduce in renal failure) or a PPI can be used to reduce the delivery of acid to the duodenum.

Parenteral nutrition

Nutritional support is very important due to the increased metabolic demands of the disease, but oral feeding should be avoided in the acute phase. Long-term enteral feeding via a feeding tube placed beyond the proximal duodenum is a preferred route of nutrition. Insulin may be required if pancreatic injury is severe.

Respiratory support

Supplemental oxygen should be administered to all but very mild cases. Hypoxia develops as a result of abdominal distension and atelectasis, impaired perfusion, fluid overload, and the involvement of the pulmonary microcirculation in the systemic inflammatory process. Close observation of oxygen saturation and arterial blood gases will detect the patient who requires ventilatory support.

Renal support

It is essential to carefully monitor urine output, fluid balance, and urea and electrolytes. Hemofiltration/dialysis is often necessary in severe cases.

Antibiotics

Prophylactic cover against organisms in the GI tract is recommended in severe attacks.

Endoscopy

Endoscopic release of calculi within the biliary system may be appropriate.

Surgery

Surgical débridement of a necrotic pancreas may be necessary in very severe cases in order to remove a persistent source of ongoing inflammation/infection. This is often guided by contrast-enhanced CT, which may also demonstrate localized collections suitable for percutaneous drainage.

Complications

The complications of severe disease can be summarized as follows:

- Local: prolonged ileus and splanchnic ischemia, pancreatic necrosis, abscess/pseudocyst, and ascites ± fistula (with resulting fluid and metabolic disturbance).
- Organ dysfunction: eg, pancreatic (eg, diabetes mellitus) and distant dysfunction. There is a spectrum of multiple organ dysfunction, most notably nosocomial infections, acute lung injury, acute renal failure, GI failure, dis-

seminated intravascular coagulation/hematological failure, hepatic failure, and refractory low output cardiac failure.

- Chronic pancreatitis, exocrine and endocrine insufficiency.

Chapter 9

Infection and inflammation

Brian Gehlbach
University of Chicago, Chicago, IL, USA

Although many critically ill patients present with the clinical signs of sepsis (eg, tachycardia, fever), in many cases a true infectious cause cannot be established. Some of these patients will exhibit signs of acute inflammation (Figure 9.1) from a noninfectious cause, such as trauma, pancreatitis, or burns. Furthermore, it is hypothesized that it is the potentially tissue-destroying elements of this systemic inflammatory response syndrome (SIRS) that are central to the subsequent evolution of multiple organ dysfunction syndrome (MODS). Consensus conferences have elaborated on these ideas, allowing

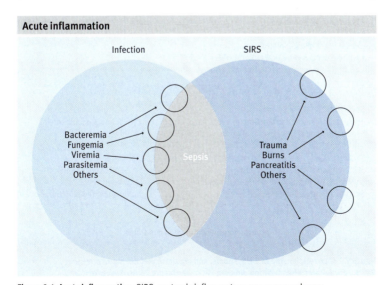

Figure 9.1 Acute inflammation. SIRS, systemic inflammatory response syndrome.

distinction between sepsis and inflammation only when a true infective element is identified (Figure 9.2).

Infection in critically ill individuals

Severe infection is not only a common cause of admission to intensive care, but also the most common complication suffered by critically ill patients. Both patient and environmental factors account for this increased susceptibility (Figure 9.3). Common sites for infection in critically ill patients are:

- the chest
- intravascular catheters ('line sepsis')
- bacteremia, unknown source
- wounds/drains
- the urinary tract
- intra-abdominal.

Hospital-acquired pneumonia

Hospital-acquired pneumonia (HAP) is defined as a pneumonia diagnosed 48 h or more after admission, which was not incubating at the time of

---

Interrelationship of SIRS, sepsis, and organ failure

SIRS: manifested by two or more of the following:
- temperature >38°C or <36°C
- heart rate >90 beats/min
- respiratory rate >20 breaths/min or $PaCO_2$ <4.3 kPa (33 mmHg)
- white cell count >12,000 cells/mm³ or <4,000 cells/mm³ or >10% immature forms

Sepsis: SIRS plus documented infection

Severe SIRS: SIRS associated with evidence of hypotension, organ dysfunction, or evidence of organ hypoperfusion (eg, confusion, oliguria, lactic acidosis)

Severe sepsis: severe SIRS plus documented infection

SIRS related shock: hypotension (systolic BP <90 mmHg or 40 mmHg <baseline) despite adequate fluid resuscitation

Septic shock: SIRS-related shock plus documented infection

Multiple organ dysfunction syndrome

Figure 9.2 Interrelationship of SIRS, sepsis, and organ failure. BP, blood pressure; $PaCO_2$, partial pressure of carbon dioxide; PaO_2, partial pressure of oxygen; SIRS, systemic inflammatory response syndrome.

Factors predisposing to infection in critically ill patients	
Patient factors	**Environmental factors**
Acute and chronic disease states	Opportunistic organisms
Tracheal intubation	Cramped bed spaces
Reduced immunocompetence	Poor hand hygiene
Malnutrition	Contaminated equipment
Multiple vascular catheters and drains	Poor compliance with basic infection control policies
Raised gastric pH	
Elderly population	
Use of (broad-spectrum) antibiotics	

Figure 9.3 Factors predisposing to infection in critically ill patients.

admission. In contrast to the hospital population as a whole (in whom urinary tract and wound infections are more frequent), it is the most common infection in the critically ill, and is associated with a mortality rate of up to 50%. Risk factors include the following:

- intubation and ventilation, as a result of cough suppression (due to necessity for sedation), repeated tracheal suction, and microaspiration of (infected) oropharyngeal contents
- impaired airway protection, due to dysfunction of the central nervous system, drugs, and nasogastric tube
- surgical factors predisposing to infection in the critically ill patient
- chronic obstructive pulmonary disease
- antibiotic therapy
- severe underlying disease
- immunosuppression
- malnutrition
- raised gastric pH (bacterial overgrowth of stomach).

Although community-acquired pathogens can cause HAP, there is a much higher incidence of infection caused by aerobic Gram-negative bacilli. This is possibly the result of overgrowth of the stomach with intestinal bacteria, or the direct vascular spread of organisms that have translocated across the intestinal wall into the circulation. Ventilator-associated pneumonia (VAP) refers to pneumonia that arises more than 48–72 h after endotracheal intubation.

Diagnosis

The clinical features used to diagnose HAP and VAP (eg, fever, leukocytosis, purulent sputum production, and new infiltrates on a chest X-ray) are unreliable in the setting of critical illness. Fever and leukocytosis are nonspecific markers of inflammation. Bacterial colonization of the respiratory tract is common, so that the presence of organisms in tracheal secretions does not necessarily represent infection. Pulmonary infiltrates on a chest X-ray can have other causes (eg, fluid overload or atelectasis). Blood cultures provide retrospective confirmation of infection, but are less commonly positive than in community-acquired pneumonia.

Sampling of sputum obtained from the distal areas of the respiratory tract using techniques that prevent contamination with the resident flora of the trachea and major bronchi helps distinguish between colonization and true infection. Such semi-quantitative methods include:

- protected specimen brushing (where >1,000 colony-forming units/mL suggests infection)
- bronchoalveolar lavage (>10,000 colony-forming units/mL suggests infection).

Patients with suspected VAP should have a lower respiratory tract specimen cultured via one of the above techniques or via endotracheal aspiration prior to administering new antimicrobial therapy.

Antibiotic therapy

In practice, treatment must often be started on the basis of the clinical circumstances, previous antibiotic therapy, urgent Gram stain of sputum, and the antibiotic policies of an individual hospital. The organisms commonly involved in HAP, along with their antibiotic sensitivities, are listed in Figures 9.4 and 9.5. Patients with HAP or VAP who do not have risk factors for multidrug-resistant (MDR) pathogens and have early onset (within the first 4 days of hospitalization) pneumonia may be treated according to the recommendations in Figure 9.4. Patients with late-onset pneumonia, or risk factors for MDR pathogens, are treated according to the recommendations in Figure 9.5. Risk factors for MDR pathogens include antimicrobial therapy in the preceding 90 days, a high frequency of antibiotic resistance in the community or hospital unit, recent hospitalization, residence in a nursing home or extended-care facility, home infusion therapy, chronic dialysis, home wound care, a family member with resistant pathogen, and immunosuppressive disease and/or therapy. Given that there is considerable variation between hospitals concerning the frequency and patterns of resistance of organisms causing nosocomial infections, the suggested regimens must be adjusted accordingly.

Empiric antibiotic therapy for HAP or VAP in patients with early onset and no known risk factors for MDR pathogens

Potential pathogen	Recommended antibiotic
Streptococcus pneumoniae	Ceftriaxone
Haemophilus influenzae	or
Meticillin-sensitive *Staphylococcus aureus*	Levofloxacin, moxifloxacin,
Antibiotic-sensitive enteric Gram-negative	or
bacilli	Ciprofloxacin
	or
	Ampicillin/sulbactam or
	ertapenem

Figure 9.4 Empiric antibiotic therapy for HAP or VAP in patients with early onset and no known risk factors for MDR pathogens. HAP, hospital-acquired pneumonia; MDR, multidrug resistant; VAP, ventilator-associated pneumonia.

Empiric antibiotic therapy for HAP or VAP in patients with late-onset disease or risk factors for MDR pathogens

Potential pathogens	Combination antibiotic therapy
Pathogens from Figure 9.4 and MDR	Antipseudomonal cephalosporin (cefepime,
pathogens	ceftazidime)
Pseudomonas aeruginosa	or
Klebsiella pneumoniae	Antipseudomonal carbepenem (imipenem or
Acinetobacter spp.	meropenem)
Meticillin-resistant *S. aureus*	or
Legionella pneumophila	β-Lactam/β-lactamase inhibitor (piperacillin
	with tazobactam)
	plus
	Antipseudomonal fluoroquinolone
	(ciprofloxacin or levofloxacin)
	or
	Aminoglycoside (amikacin, gentamicin, or
	tobramycin)
	plus
	Linezolid or vancomycin

Figure 9.5 Empiric antibiotic therapy for HAP or VAP in patients with late-onset disease or risk factors for MDR pathogens. HAP, hospital-acquired penumonia; MDR, multidrug resistant; VAP, ventilator-associated pneumonia.

Nosocomial bacteremia

Nosocomial bacteremias are associated with the following primary sources of infection:

- intravascular catheters
- pneumonia

Management of nosocomial bacteremia

Organism	Therapy
Coagulase-negative staphylococci	Remove suspect line; vancomycin
Staphylococcus aureus	Identify source and treat if possible; nafcillin; gentamicin or rifampin may be added in severe infections; erythromycin and cefazolin also have anti-staphylococcal activity; vancomycin if meticillin resistant
Streptococcus spp.	Benzylpenicillin (but ampicillin + gentamicin for *Enterococcus faecalis*)
Gram-negative organisms	Identify source (chest, abdomen, etc); antibiotic options include:
Enterobacteriaceae	Gentamicin or cefotaxime
Salmonella typhi	Ciprofloxacin
Pseudomonas aeruginosa	Gentamicin + piperacillin, ciprofloxacin, aztreonam, imipenem
	The choice depends on the clinical circumstances and the identity of the organism. Metronidazole should be added if intra-abdominal sepsis is the likely source
Fungi	Amphotericin, caspofungin, or voriconazole

Figure 9.6 Management of nosocomial bacteremia.

- urinary tract
- wounds/drains
- intra-abdominal
- endocarditis.

Of these foci, intravascular catheters are the most important, accounting for the prevalence of Gram-positive organisms in positive blood cultures in critically ill patients. So-called 'line sepsis' is particularly common with central venous catheters, especially when inserted in less than optimal conditions (eg, as an emergency in the resuscitation room), if the placement is difficult and/or performed by an inexperienced operator, and when placed in the femoral vein. There is no clear evidence that duration of residence in itself increases the risk of bacteremia. The organisms implicated in nosocomial bacteremia are listed in Figure 9.6, along with suggested management.

Other causes of sepsis in the intensive care unit

Intra-abdominal sepsis

It is important to identify and treat the cause of sepsis. Ampicillin (*Enterococcus faecalis*), gentamicin (Gram-negative organisms), and metronidazole (anaerobes) are traditional combinations. A second or third-generation cephalosporin may be substituted for gentamicin. Altered flora due to previous broad-spectrum antibiotic therapy may require additional pseudomonal coverage (eg, piperacillin).

Necrotizing fasciitis
Mixed aerobic and anaerobic organisms (ie, group A streptococci) are involved in necrotizing fasciitis. A third-generation cephalosporin, gentamicin, and metronidazole, or benzylpenicillin is recommended in cases of streptococcal infection.

Urinary tract infections
Urinary tract infections are unusual in critically ill catheterized patients. Antibiotics should not be given unless there are systemic signs of sepsis. Gram-negative organisms such as *E. coli*, *Proteus* spp. or *Klebsiella* spp. are most common. Treatment options depend on sensitivities but include trimethoprim, ampicillin, ciprofloxacin, or aminoglycoside.

Meningitis
Neisseria meningitidis, the Gram-negative bacterium known for its role in meningitis, is best treated with ceftriaxone. It can also be used to treat the Gram-negative bacterium *Hemophilus influenzae*. In the case of *Streptococcus pneumoniae* cefotaxime or ceftriaxone are recommended, and vancomycin should be added pending sensitivities in regions with penicillin- or cephalosporin-resistant pneumococci.

Brain abscess
A brain abscess should be managed with cefotaxime and metronidazole at high doses.

Endocarditis
The following antibiotics are recommended in the treatment of the following organisms in endocarditis:
- *Streptococcus viridans*: benzylpenicillin + gentamicin
- *Enterococcus faecalis*: resistance frequent; potential agents include benzyl-pencillin, ampicillin, gentamicin, vancomycin
- Meticillin-sensitive *S. aureus* (MSSA) (native valve): nafcillin + gentamicin
- Meticillin-resistant *S. aureus* (MRSA) (native valve): vancomycin ± rifampin
- MSSA (prosthetic valve): nafcillin + rifampin + gentamicin
- MRSA (prosthetic valve): vancomycin + rifampin + gentamicin
- coagulase-negative staphylococci: vancomycin.

Anthrax

Bacillus anthracis is a Gram-positive, aerobic, spore-forming bacillus. It has an increasing relevance due to its potential use in biologic warfare. Inhalational anthrax exhibits prodrome of flu-like illness with fever, malaise, dry cough, chest discomfort, and myalgias. The second phase is characterized by hemorrhagic thoracic lymphadenitis and mediastinitis, shock, and rapid progression to death within 24–48 h. Presumptive diagnosis is by clinical suspicion, radiological findings of a widened mediastinum, and a Gram stain smear of infected body fluid. Notifying Centers for Disease Control and Prevention (CDC) for confirmation and control is mandatory. Cutaneous and gastrointestinal presentations exist; *Anthrax meningitis* is associated with a very high mortality, and initial therapy is ciprofloxacin (± penicillin).

Commonly used antibiotics

The most widely used antibiotics are the penicillins, cephalosporins, β-lactams, aminoglycosides, and other antibiotics such as ciprofloxacin and vancomycin, to name but a few. It is important to consult a dosing guide to adjust for renal impairment.

Penicillins

Benzylpenicillin

Benzylpenicillin is the first choice treatment of infections due to β-hemolytic streptococci, pneumococci, meningococci, clostridia, and pasturellae. Reduced sensitivity of pneumococci to benzylpenicillin has been reported. Benzylpenicillin is inactivated by penicillinase-producing organisms. It has variable gut absorption, and there is a risk of convulsions if given in high doses (particularly in renal failure). As with all penicillins, it must not be given intrathecally due to a risk of fatal encephalopathy. A parenteral dose of 1–3 MU should be administered every 4 h.

Ampicillin

Ampicillin has a broader Gram-negative activity than benzylpenicillin, but it is inferior against organisms sensitive to the latter, and is inactivated by penicillinase. Most staphylococci (eg, 50% of *E. coli* and 20% of *Hemophilus influenzae*) are resistant to ampicillin. It is well excreted into bile and urine. A parenteral dose of 0.5–1 g every 6 h is recommended.

Nafcillin

MRSA is endemic in many hospitals and nursing homes, and nafcillin is a penicillinase-resistant penicillin used for the treatment of *S. aureus* infections. A parenteral dose of 1.5–3 g every 6 h is recommended.

Piperacillin

Piperacillin is a broad-spectrum penicillin that should be reserved for the treatment of serious infections where *Pseudomonas* spp. are likely (eg, immunosuppressed individuals), and also with extended enteric Gram-negative activity. It should be combined with an aminoglycoside to prevent the emergence of resistant strains, and can be combined with a penicillinase inhibitor (eg, tazobactam). A parenteral dose of 2–4 g every 4–6 h is recommended.

Cephalosporins

These are broad-spectrum antibiotics; 5% of penicillin-sensitive patients exhibit cross-sensitivity to cephalosporins. Below is an outline of some of the antibiotics used most commonly in the intensive care unit for treating infections.

Cefazolin

Cefazolin is a first-generation cephalosporin. It is stable against many penicillinases, and therefore exhibits useful anti-staphylococcal activity. It is commonly used for surgical prophylaxis, and a parenteral dose of 0.5–2 g every 8 h is advised.

Cefuroxime

Cefuroxime is a second-generation cephalosporin, active against a broad range of Gram-positive and Gram-negative organisms, but not enterococci, *Pseudomonas* spp., or anaerobes. It is also stable with many penicillinases. A parenteral dose of 0.75–1.5 g every 8 h is advised.

Cefotaxime

Cefotaxime is a third-generation cephalosporin and has a broader Gram-negative activity than cefuroxime, but it is less active against Gram-positive organisms such as *S. aureus*. It has some anti-anaerobic activity. It should not be used if pseudomonal infection is likely. There is a significant risk of pseudomembranous colitis and superinfection with resistant Gram-negative organisms or fungi. A parenteral dose of 1–2 g every 8 h is recommended.

Ceftazidime

Ceftazidime is active against the same organisms as cefuroxime, but its activity is extended to pseudomonal species. A parenteral dose of 1–2 g every 8 h is advised.

Other β-lactams
Imipenem

Imipenem is a very broad-spectrum antibiotic, active against many aerobic and anaerobic Gram-positive and Gram-negative bacteria, including most penicillinase producers. It is presented in combination with cilastin, which inhibits its renal metabolism. It should be reserved for problem infections, and pseudomonal resistance may develop quickly. A parenteral dose of 0.5–1 g every 6 h is recommended.

Aztreonam

Aztreonam shows good activity against Gram-negative organisms, including *Pseudomonas* spp. A parenteral dose of 1–2 g every 8 h is recommended.

Aminoglycosides

These are bactericidal against some Gram-positive and many Gram-negative organisms. They must be given parenterally and can be ototoxic (particularly in combination with other drugs such as furosemide) and nephrotoxic, and may interfere with neuromuscular transmission. They are traditionally given every 8–12 h, although once-daily administration is now recommended in most patient groups; drug levels should be monitored.

Gentamicin

Gentamicin is the drug of choice in serious infections arising from Gram-negative organisms, with activity against *Pseudomonas* spp. It also has useful activity against *S. aureus*. It has no anaerobic activity and no intrinsic activity against streptococci, but it is synergistic with penicillin for the treatment of bacterial endocarditis. A parenteral dose of 1–1.5 mg/kg every 8 h, or 7 mg/kg (intravenous over 1 h) once daily is recommended.

Amikacin

Amikacin is reserved for gentamicin-resistant Gram-negative organisms. A parenteral dose of 7.5 mg/kg every 12 h is recommended.

Other antibiotics
Ciprofloxacin

Ciprofloxacin is a broad-spectrum quinolone antibiotic, with particularly good Gram-negative activity, including against *Pseudomonas* spp. Its activity against Gram-positive organisms is modest, with little activity against *S. aureus*. It has little anaerobic activity, but is well absorbed orally. It is used to treat infections of the respiratory and urinary tracts, particularly in patients with resistant organisms that have emerged during previous antibiotic therapy. There is a risk of convulsions, which is increased in patients with hepatorenal impairment, or those receiving nonsteroidal anti-inflammatory drugs. A parenteral dose of 200–400 mg every 12 h is recommended.

Vancomycin

Vancomycin inhibits cell wall synthesis. It is the drug of choice in the treatment of MRSA and coagulase-negative staphylococci that are resistant to meticillin. However, it is nephrotoxic and ototoxic, and serum levels must be monitored carefully. Rapid intravenous administration causes cardiovascular collapse. Orally, it is used to treat pseudomembranous colitis. A parenteral dose of 1 g every 12 h, reduced in renal impairment according to plasma levels, is recommended.

Erythromycin

Erythromycin is a useful, but less potent, alternative to penicillin and nafcillin. It is the drug of choice in Legionnaire's disease, and infections with *Mycoplasma pneumoniae* and *Campylobacter* spp. Its prokinetic properties are useful in patients with gastric stasis. A parenteral dose of 500 mg to 1 g every 6 h is recommended.

Metronidazole

Metronidazole is active only against obligate anaerobes and protozoa (eg, *Trichomonas*, *Giardia*, *Entamoeba* spp.). It is the first-line treatment for pseudomembranous colitis. A parenteral dose of 500 mg every 8 h is recommended.

Trimethoprim and sulfamethoxazole

Trimethoprim (TMP) and sulfamethoxazole (SMX) are used in prophylaxis and in the treatment of pneumocystis pneumonia in patients who are immunocompromised. A parenteral dose of 160–240 mg TMP and 800–1200 mg SMX every 6–12 h is recommended.

Rifampin

Rifampin is a broad-spectrum antibiotic used in the treatment of tuberculosis and severe staphylococcal infections, and as prophylaxis in contacts of meningococcal and hemophilus meningitis. A parenteral dose of 0.6–1.2 g daily in two to four divided doses is recommended.

Antiviral agents

Aciclovir

Aciclovir is active against herpes simplex types 1 and 2, varicella-zoster, and, when administered in high doses, the Epstein–Barr virus. It is the drug of choice in the treatment of herpes encephalitis, and disseminated herpes and zoster infections in the immunocompromised patient. A parenteral dose of 5–10 mg/kg every 8 h is recommended.

Ganciclovir

Ganciclovir is used in the treatment of life-threatening cytomegalovirus (CMV) infections; however, it causes anemia and neutropenia. A parenteral dose of 5 mg/kg every 12 h is recommended.

Foscarnet

Foscarnet is used in the treatment of aciclovir-resistant mucocutaneous herpes simplex infections in immunocompromised patients and for CMV retinitis. Significant side effects include fever, metabolic disturbances, gastro-intestinal upset, anemia, and granulocytopenia. Intravenous adult doses for aciclovir-resistant HSV infection is 40 mg/kg every 8–12 h, with adjustment for creatinine clearance.

Valganciclovir

Valganciclovir is a newer oral antiviral agent used to treat CMV retinitis in patients with acquired immune deficiency syndrome and to prevent CMV infection in patients undergoing solid organ transplantation. Significant adverse reactions include fever, gastrointestinal upset, granulocytopenia, and anemia. The adult dose for the prevention of CMV disease following transplantation is 900 mg orally once daily (with food) beginning within 10 days of transplantation until 100 days post-transplant.

Antifungal agents

Amphotericin

Amphotericin is the drug of choice in life-threatening systemic fungal infections, but there is a high risk of hypersensitivity and nephrotoxicity. Liposomal preparations are less toxic but expensive. A 1 mg test dose, followed by 250 mg/kg daily, gradually increasing to a maximum of 1.5 mg/kg per day in severe infections, is recommended.

Fluconazole

Fluconazole is a less toxic alternative to amphotericin in the treatment of some candida infections. A parenteral dose of 400 mg initially, followed by 200–400 mg daily, is recommended.

Flucytosine

Flucytosine is active in systemic candida and cryptococcal infections, and is used in combination with amphotericin to prevent resistance. A parenteral dose of 50 mg/kg every 6 h is recommended.

Voriconazole

Voriconazole is a triazole with activity against both *Aspergillus* and *Candida* spp. The dosing varies according to indication.

Caspofungin

Caspofungin is the option for treatment of infections caused by *Candida* and *Aspergillus* spp., as well as for intra-abdominal abscesses and febrile neutropenia. A dosage of 70 mg i.v. on day 1, followed by 50 mg i.v daily thereafter, is usually administered.

Chapter 10

Hematologic emergencies

Imre Noth
University of Chicago, Chicago, IL, USA

Sickle cell disorders

The sickle cell disorders (Figure 10.1) are a group of inherited conditions, characterized by the presence of a structurally and functionally abnormal form of hemoglobin (Hb) called hemoglobin S (HbS). The clinical consequences range from the benign heterozygous condition of sickle cell trait (HbAS) to the potentially life-threatening conditions of homozygous sickle cell disease (HbSS). Compound heterozygous conditions, in which one HbS gene is combined with genes coding for other structural variants of hemoglobin (eg, hemoglobins C, D, or E) or with genes responsible for different forms of thalassemia, have a variable presentation.

Incidence

There is a high incidence among black populations in central Africa, the West Indies, and North America, with a lower incidence in the Indian subcontinent and the Mediterranean.

Pathophysiology

Normal adult hemoglobin (HbA) is made up of four polypeptide chains, two α and two β subunits. HbS differs from HbA as a result of the substitution of valine for glutamic acid at position 6 of the β chain, resulting in a molecule that, although soluble when oxygenated, crystallizes out of solution when deoxygenated to distort erythrocytes and give them their characteristic sickle shape. Sickled erythrocytes obstruct the microcirculation and thereby lead to tissue ischemia and infarction. The principal cause of sickling is a reduction in tissue oxygen tension (PO_2), so that crises are induced by hypoxia, hypothermia, dehydration, acidosis, and infection. In sickle cell trait, 20–40%

Sickle cell disorders

Disorder	β subunit genotype	Clinical features
Sickle cell trait	AS	Benign; problems only in extreme circumstances, such as profound hypoxia, hypothermia
Sickle cell disease	SS	Hemolytic anemia; infection; chronic pain; cardiopulmonary failure
Sickle cell hemoglobin C disease	SC	Mild anemia and thrombotic episodes
Sickle cell hemoglobin D disease	SD	Similar to sickle cell anemia
Sickle cell β-thalassemia	Sβthal	Variable according to the severity of the thalassemia

Figure 10.1 Sickle cell disorders.

of the total hemoglobin is HbS, the remainder being HbA. Significant sickling does not occur until the tissue PO_2 has fallen to 2.5 kPa (20 mmHg). In contrast, in HbSS 95–98% of hemoglobin is HbS and sickling occurs at tissue PO_2 of 5.5 kPa (40 mmHg) or less.

Laboratory diagnosis
Hemoglobin solubility tests such as the Sickledex test identify the presence of HbS, but do not distinguish between sickle cell trait and sickle cell disease. Hemoglobin electrophoresis provides the definitive diagnosis, demonstrating the relative proportions of HbA and HbS, as well as revealing the presence of other variants such as HbC.

Sickle cell trait
A benign condition in which significant sickling occurs only under the most extreme conditions (eg, hypothermic cardiopulmonary bypass, the extreme hypoxia of high altitude). Affected individuals have a normal hemoglobin concentration and hematologic profile.

Sickle cell disease
The clinical features of the disease are those of acute exacerbations (ie, crises) superimposed upon a progressive chronic disease state. The striking variability of the severity of the disease is a result of differences in the levels of fetal hemoglobin. Features of chronic disease include the following:
• Chronic hemolytic anemia – red cell life span is 15–25 days, Hb 6–8 g/dL; other abnormal hematologic indices include a reticulocytosis, mild elevations

of the white cell and platelet counts, and the characteristic peripheral blood film appearances of polychromatophilic red cells, Howell–Jolly bodies, and sickled erythrocytes.

- Cor pulmonale – due to recurrent infection and pulmonary embolic disease.
- Progressive small vessel disease – renal failure, cerebrovascular disease, asplenism, increasing susceptibility to infection, aseptic necrosis of bones (particularly femoral and humeral heads).
- Iron overload from multiple transfusions.

Acute crises

Different forms of acute crisis are recognized, and presentations frequently vary; these are summarized below:

- Thrombotic – obstruction of small vessels by clumps of sickled red cells results in ischemic pain and organ dysfunction. Long bone pain, with underlying marrow ischemia, and abdominal pain, which may be associated with an ileus, may also present. Acute chest syndrome occurs in approximately 30% of patients and is the leading cause of death in patients with sickle cell disease. It usually presents with a new pulmonary infiltrate, fever, respiratory symptoms, or chest pain. Moreover, while up to a third of patients do not have radiological changes, progressive hypoxemia may still be present. Some patients progress to acute respiratory distress syndrome and require aggressive management with early intubation and mechanical ventilation. An infection is rarely identified, but often presumed. Neurologic dysfunction, such as transient ischemic attacks, and cerebral hemorrhage may also manifest, and may be accompanied by an increased rate of hemolysis.
- Infective – repeated episodes of splenic infarction significantly impair antibacterial host defenses. Patients present with septicemia (common pathogens include *Streptococcus pneumoniae*, *Hemophilus influenzae*) and/or osteomyelitis (commonly *Staphylococcus aureus*, but occasionally *Salmonella typhimurium*).
- Aplastic – episodes of temporary bone marrow failure, possibly related to intercurrent viral illness.
- Sequestration – occurs mainly in children. Acute sequestration of sickled erythrocytes in spleen and liver. Patients present with life-threatening anemia, abdominal pain, and hepatosplenomegaly.

Management of acute crises

Early intervention in crises not only shortens and relieves patient discomfort but reduces the incidence of complications in the long term:

- General measures – regardless of the nature of the crisis, adequate hydration and oxygenation should be maintained in order to limit any sickling process (intravenous fluids, ≥3 L/24 h, and supplemental oxygen as guided by continuous oxygen saturation measurements). Patients should be closely monitored for the development of a life-threatening sequestration crisis by daily or twice-daily examination for evolving hepatosplenomegaly, along with daily measurement of hematocrit and reticulocyte count.
- Infection – fever provokes sickling, so prompt investigation and vigorous, and sometimes blind, treatment of infection may be necessary. Septicemia should be treated with an intravenous cephalosporin with activity against pneumococci and *H. influenzae* (eg, cefotaxime 1–2 g every 8 h, children 50 mg/kg every 8 h). Osteomyelitis should be treated with a fluoroquinolone in an effort to cover *Salmonella* spp. Other intravenous choices include nafcillin/oxacillin 1–2 g every 6 h (children: under 2 years 25% adult dose, 2–10 years 50% adult dose), together with an aminoglycoside.
- Analgesia – intravenous opiates are often required.
- Transfusion – Hb should be maintained at approximately 10 g/dL. Exchange transfusion, aimed at reducing the HbS levels to less than 30%, should be considered in the event of serious pulmonary interstitial emphysema 'acute chest syndrome' or cerebral thrombotic crises.
- Anticoagulation – indicated in serious thrombotic crises.

Transfusion reactions

A transfusion reaction can be defined as any untoward reaction that occurs as a consequence of infusion of blood or one of its components. The following ill effects of blood transfusion will be considered here:

- consequences of massive transfusion
- acute hemolytic transfusion reactions
- nonhemolytic allergic/anaphylactoid reactions.

Massive transfusion

Massive transfusion can be arbitrarily defined as either transfusion with more than 10% blood volume in 10 min (or less) or transfusion with more than 50% blood volume during the course of surgery. The consequences of a massive transfusion depend on:

- the differences between stored and endogenous blood

- hypovolemic shock, in particular splanchnic ischemia
- the nature of the primary pathology (eg, trauma).

The important ways in which stored blood differs from endogenous blood, and the clinical consequences that result, are discussed and listed below:

- temperature
- clotting factors and platelets
- tissue oxygenation
- microaggregates
- acid–base balance
- electrolytes
- red cell survival.

Temperature

Blood for transfusion is stored at 4°C. Rapid transfusion of large volumes of poorly warmed blood causes hypothermia, which can lead to:

- impaired clotting
- dysrhythmias and myocardial depression
- shivering and increased oxygen requirements
- delayed drug clearance
- increased blood viscosity
- interference with citrate and lactate metabolism
- increased intracellular potassium release
- a shift of the oxyhemoglobin dissociation curve to the left.

Efficient warming devices should be used when transfusing more than 2 units of blood.

Clotting factors and platelets

Stored blood becomes depleted of plasma clotting factors (particularly factors V and VIII) and platelets within days of donation. Citrate is added to chelate calcium and thereby inhibits coagulation. Hemostatic failure is a common consequence of massive blood transfusion, for several reasons:

- dilution of endogenous clotting factors with synthetic colloid or human albumin solutions
- reduced synthesis/release of clotting factors (hepatic ischemia)
- chelation of calcium by citrate
- thrombocytopenia
- hypothermia and disseminated intravascular coagulation (DIC).

As a rule of thumb, 2 units of fresh frozen plasma (FFP) and 10 mL 10% calcium gluconate should be given per 4 units of blood.

Tissue oxygenation

Stored blood is cold and depleted of 2,3-diphosphoglycerate (2,3-DPG). Hypothermia and reduced 2,3-DPG shift the oxyhemoglobin dissociation curve to the left, resulting in reduced tissue oxygen delivery.

Microaggregates

White cells and platelets clump during storage to form aggregates 100–200 mm in diameter. Accumulation of microaggregates in the microcirculation is associated with acute lung injury and hypoxemia, generalized tissue ischemia, and DIC and complement activation.

The use of filters to remove microaggregates is still disputed, although many advocate their use when more than 1 L of blood is transfused.

Acid–base balance

Blood stored for 3 weeks has a pH of 6.7, due to the accumulation of lactate and the addition of citrate as an anticoagulant. Massive transfusion is frequently associated with a metabolic acidosis, and potential causes include a lactic acidosis secondary to hypovolemic shock, or transfused acids, such as lactate and citrate, where the latter is usually metabolized to bicarbonate in the liver.

Electrolytes

An increasing proportion of erythrocytes lyze during storage, leading to an increase in the extracellular potassium (K^+) concentration to 25 mmol/L after 3 weeks. Extracellular sodium (Na^+) concentration also rises to 150–160 mol/L. The risk of hyperkalemia following massive transfusion has probably been overstated, with many of the lyzed cells recovering once they have rewarmed to reaccumulate K^+. Indeed, this may lead to hypokalemia as the patient recovers over the following 24 h.

Red cell survival

As noted above, erythrocytes gradually lyze during storage. Free hemoglobin and its breakdown products in the circulation accelerate oxidant-mediated injury, and may thereby contribute to multiple organ dysfunction syndrome following massive transfusion. Subsequent metabolism of hemoglobin leads to jaundice.

Acute hemolytic transfusion reactions

The clinical features of acute intravascular hemolysis are listed below, and result from the release of hemoglobin, potassium, and other red cell contents into the plasma. Causes include:

- immunological – ABO incompatibility, hemolysins, multiple donor incompatibility
- transfusion with stored blood that is already hemolyzed – prolonged storage (after 35 days storage only 70% of transfused red cells will survive for 24 h or more), thermal injury (freezing or heat).

The most dangerous reactions are the acute immunologic hemolytic reactions to red cell transfusion, most of which are due to ABO incompatibility and are thus preventable. Other antibodies are rarer, and occur only after previous exposure to foreign antigens, or are active only at temperatures below 37°C.

Clinical features
Presentation is variable, and may manifest in the following ways:
- agitation
- back/abdominal pain
- rigors
- hypotension and cardiovascular collapse
- DIC
- renal failure
- anemia.

Management
Successful management of acute hemolytic transfusion reactions involves cessation of transfusion and keeping the remainder for subsequent investigation. Ensuring a brisk diuresis (eg, 0.9% saline + loop diuretic) is important, as well as supporting the cardiorespiratory system.

Nonhemolytic transfusion reactions
These are a complex array of immunological phenomena, ranging from true allergic-type reactions to antigenic components of blood products to nonimmunological stimulation of other aspects of the immune system (eg, direct activation of complement or histamine release). A clinical grading scheme for such reactions has been proposed and is shown in Figure 10.2.

Management
As with acute hemolytic transfusion, the management of nonhemolytic transfusions also involves stopping transfusion, and keeping the remainder for investigation. However, antihistamines, bronchodilators, and circulatory support are also necessary.

Grading scheme for nonhemolytic transfusion reactions

I	Skin manifestations such as pruritiś, rash, urticaria
II	Mild-to-moderate hypotension, gastrointestinal upset, and respiratory distress
III	Severe hypotension/shock, bronchospasm
IV	Cardiorespiratory arrest

Figure 10.2 Grading scheme for nonhemolytic transfusion reactions.

Disseminated intravascular coagulation

Normal hemostasis depends upon a number of interrelated responses, such as vasoconstriction, formation of a platelet plug, fibrin clot formation, and controlled fibrinolysis to limit the extent of the coagulum. Formation of a fibrin clot (Figure 10.3) is the result of the activation of an amplifying cascade of plasma proteolytic enzymes, initiated by contact stimulation from the vascular endothelium and platelet plug (intrinsic system) or the release of thromboplastins from damaged tissues (extrinsic system). These two initiating limbs impinge upon a final common pathway of activation of factor X and the subsequent conversion of prothrombin to thrombin. Thrombin catalyzes the formation of fibrin monomers from fibrinogen, which then polymerize to form a fibrin clot. Thrombin also promotes fibrinolysis by converting plasminogen into plasmin.

Formation of a fibrin clot

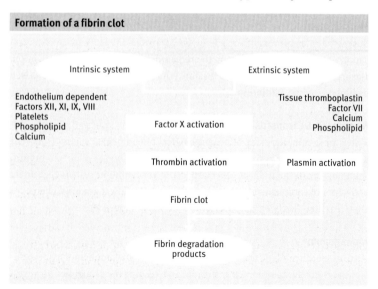

Figure 10.3 Formation of a fibrin clot.

The activated system is controlled by inhibitory factors such as antithrombin III, which irreversibly inhibits factor X.

DIC is a loosely defined syndrome in which the processes of platelet plugging, coagulation, and fibrinolysis are inappropriately activated and the normal inhibitory control mechanisms are lost. It thereby results in:

- consumption of procoagulant proteins and platelets
- accumulation of fibrin degradation products (FDPs), which are themselves anticoagulant
- an apparently paradoxical combination of intravascular fibrin deposition (leading to tissue ischemia and organ failure) and abnormal (and sometimes uncontrollable) hemorrhage.

Causes

The causes of DIC vary and can range from a bacterial infection to heat stroke; these and other causes are listed below:

- infection – bacterial, especially Gram-negative organisms, viral (eg, cytomegalovirus), protozoal (eg, malaria)
- systemic inflammatory response syndrome – hypovolemic shock, trauma, burns, acute lung injury
- pregnancy – abruption, eclampsia, amniotic fluid embolism, retained products of conception, sepsis
- malignancy – disseminated, leukemias
- miscellaneous – incompatible blood transfusion, massive intravascular hemolysis, pulmonary embolism, fat embolism, heat stroke, envenomation, antigen–antibody complexes.

Clinical features

The cause of DIC often dominates the overall clinical picture. Bleeding may be particularly problematic in the acute phase, and ranges from easy bruising, gingival bleeding, epistaxis, and excessive bleeding from wounds and puncture sites to the uncontrollable and life-threatening hemorrhage seen in obstetric patients. Hypotension is out of proportion to blood loss, and may be the result of the myocardial depressant action of FDPs. Microvascular thrombosis is more common in the chronic phase, during which the levels of clotting factors and platelets may be normal, representing a balance between increased production and consumption. Organ dysfunction is multifactorial (ie, primary causes, hypotension, microvascular thrombosis, etc.), and may be due to renal failure, adrenal hemorrhage, cerebral hemorrhage, or digital ischemia.

Laboratory diagnosis

Laboratory tests will often reveal that the patient has thrombocytopenia, with 90% of patients having a platelet count that is less than $150,000/mm^3$. Prolonged prothrombin and partial thromboplastin test times are also valid diagnostic tools. Hypofibrinogenemia (<160 mg/dL) and evidence of fibrinolysis (eg, FDPs >10 mg/L, elevated D-dimers, and shortened euglobin clot lysis time) are also indicators. Antithrombin III, with less than 60% normal activity, and red cell fragmentation on blood film due to microangiopathic hemolysis may be the only abnormality in chronic DIC states.

Differential diagnoses

Coagulopathy associated with liver failure and vaso-occlusive disease states (eg, sickle cell disease) form part of the differential diagnosis. Thrombotic thrombocytopenic purpura, reduced elimination of FDPs (eg, renal failure), and systemic lupus erythematosus are also indicators for DIC.

Management

Treatment with coagulation factors, platelets, and other blood products is appropriate in patients with significant bleeding or a risk thereof. Treatment of the cause is vital.

Clotting factors can be used to restore fibrinogen levels to 100 mg/dL. FFP contains most of the pro- and anticoagulant factors in plasma, and is the standard first-line treatment for bleeding complications, with an initial dose of 12–15 mL/kg.

Cryoprecipitate requires a more concentrated preparation, rich in factor VIII and fibrinogen. It is a useful adjunct to FFP therapy to boost fibrinogen levels, and is best given in 5–10 units.

In the case of platelet transfusion, some practitioners advocate maintaining a platelet count that is higher than $50,000/mm^3$, or higher if the patient is uremic. A 1 unit transfusion increases the platelet count by $5,000–10,000/mm^3$.

Inhibitory factors are used to switch off the coagulation cascade, and include heparin, endogenous inhibitors, and activated C protein. The use of heparin is controversial, particularly in the acute hemorrhagic phase, and it is best to start with low doses (eg, 5–10 IU/kg per h). Its use is also more appropriate in chronic DIC, particularly when intravascular thrombosis is more extensive. Endogenous inhibitors (eg, antithrombin III) are present in FFP. A rationale also exists for the use of activated protein C but clinical and published experience with this agent, for this indication, is limited.

All antifibrinolytics increase the risk of thrombosis. Aprotinin is a serine protease inhibitor that has an established use in open heart surgery where it is used to reduce fibrinolysis and blood loss. A loading dose of 2,000,000 units followed by 500,000 units/h is recommended. Fresh blood transfusions may be of value in cases where there is torrential obstetric hemorrhage.

Chapter 11

Nutritional support

John Kress
University of Chicago, Chicago, IL, USA

Background

Cachexia is a common consequence of critical illness, and is characterized by marked muscle breakdown. It correlates with an increased susceptibility to infection, prolonged ventilatory requirements, and mortality. Causes include the following:

- pre-existing malnutrition prior to admission to the intensive care unit (ICU)
- hypercatabolic response to critical illness
- delayed introduction of nutritional support
- immobilization.

The hypercatabolic response that accompanies severe trauma, burns, sepsis, pancreatitis, etc differs significantly from the normal physiologic response to starvation (Figure 11.1).

Nutritional requirements

Energy

The total calorie intake should be approximately equivalent to normal resting energy requirements (ie, 25–30 kcal/kg per day), and for parenteral feeding regimens approximately one-third of this should be given as fat. Patients who are very hypercatabolic (eg, with severe burns) may require more than this; however, in general an excess of calories should be avoided.

Nitrogen

Nitrogen intake should be 1–2 g protein/kg per day (this should be reduced in cases of renal failure to minimize uremia). Approximately 150 kcal of non-protein energy source are required per gram of nitrogen to permit satisfactory protein synthesis. Glutamine supplementation (≥25 g/day) may help maintain

Normal starvation versus hypercatabolic response to critical illness	
Starvation	**Hypercatabolic response to critical illness**
Reduced basal metabolic rate, reduced calorie requirements	Increased basal metabolic rate, calorie requirements. Increased secretion of 'stress' hormones (catecholamines, ortisol, etc) and cytokines
Fat becomes the principal non-carbohydrate energy source as lipolysis is stimulated by a fall in insulin and rise in glucagon	Impaired capacity to use carbohydrate and fat as energy source, resulting in an increased protein breakdown as alternative energy source
Protein and lean body mass are preserved until late into the starvation period	Massive nitrogen losses from the breakdown of muscle protein (nitrogen loss can approach 30 g per day, equivalent to 800 g muscle)
The restoration of adequate nutritional support leads to rapid resumption of an anabolic state	Catabolic state not reversed by resumption of adequate nutrition. Hyperalimentation may precipitate its own problems (lipemia, liver dysfunction, metabolic acidosis)

Figure 11.1 Normal starvation versus hypercatabolic response to critical illness.

muscle bulk. It is estimated that 1.25 g protein is equivalent to 0.2 g nitrogen or 1.5 g amino acids.

Other requirements

Additional requirements include:

- all water- and fat-soluble vitamins
- daily requirements of Na^+, K^+, Ca^{2+}, Mg^{2+}, PO_4^{3-}
- patients on long-term total parenteral nutrition (TPN) will also require supplementation with Fe^{2+}, Cu^{2+}, Zn^{2+}, Mn^{2+}
- immunonutrition, supplements of glutamine, arginine, RNA, and ω-3 fatty acids may boost immune function, although the effect on patient outcome remains unclear.

Timing

With the exception of previously well-nourished patients who will resume eating within a few days, nutritional support should start as soon as possible. The current recommendation is to start feeding within 24–48 hours of ICU admission; however, this continues to be an area of ongoing research.

Enteral nutrition

Enteral administration is considered to be the preferred mode of nutritional support and its advantages are as follows:

- It avoids the harmful effects of parenteral nutrition (eg, complications of line insertion, line sepsis, the immunosuppressive effects of intravenous lipids).

- It protects the stomach against peptic ulceration, and avoids the need for other measures such as H_2-receptor blockade.
- It helps to maintain integrity of the intestinal mucosa and gut-associated lymphoid tissue, and potentially may be able to reduce bacterial translocation.
- It is associated with a lower incidence of nosocomial infection.

Administration

A number of proprietary enteral feeds are available; 2 L will provide approximately 2,000 kcal, 75 g protein, and most of the normal daily requirements of electrolytes, vitamins, and trace elements. A daily rest period is also important as it allows restoration of gastric pH. Methods of administration include:

- Nasogastric tube – a fine-bore tube is more comfortable but does not allow aspiration to monitor absorption; larger nasogastric tubes promote gastroesophageal incompetence and possibly ulceration.
- Nasojejunal tube – overcomes gastric stasis.
- Percutaneous gastrostomy/jejunostomy – endoscopic or surgical placement is required; however, it is particularly helpful in patients requiring longer term enteral nutritional support. There may also be fewer problems with gastroesophageal reflux.

The utility of enriched enteral diets in the management of critically ill patients is controversial. One study reported a survival benefit in patients with severe sepsis who received a diet enriched with eicosapentaenoic acid, γ-linolenic acid, and antioxidant vitamins, and there is ongoing research in this area.

Failure to absorb an enteral feed is usually a result of poor gastric emptying rather than intestinal ileus, and therefore can be overcome by jejunal delivery. Factors contributing to gastric ileus include abdominal surgery, opioids, dopamine, electrolyte disturbances, to name but a few. Prokinetic agents such as erythromycin and metoclopramide (10 mg i.v. every 8 hours) may help maintain gastric motility, but are contraindicated if there is mechanical intestinal obstruction.

Complications

Diarrhea

Diarrhea is a troublesome and common complication, but not usually an indication to stop enteral nutrition. Other causes, such as *Clostridium difficile* infection, should be excluded as should overflow. Diarrhea can be treated cautiously with antimotility agents such as loperamide.

Gastroesophageal reflux and aspiration

Nasogastric intubation impairs lower esophageal sphincter function. Subsequent aspiration of potentially infected gastric contents is particularly likely in patients with poor airway protective reflexes (eg, sedation, neurologic injury), even in the presence of a cuffed endotracheal or tracheostomy tube.

Parenteral nutrition

Although TPN is indicated when enteral administration is inappropriate or has failed, the value of brief periods (eg, <1 week) of TPN is uncertain.

Feeding regimens

Daily energy and nitrogen requirements, discussed earlier, need to be modified in the case of parenteral nutrition, as follows:

- Nitrogen is given in the form of amino acids, at least 25% of which should be essential amino acids. Glutamine supplements may help preserve muscle mass and support immunocompetence.
- Energy is delivered as a combination of glucose and fat, the latter making up approximately one-third of the total calorie intake.
- Fat is delivered as a proprietary 10 or 20% emulsion of soya bean oil in glycerol and egg phosphatides. This has a higher calorific value than glucose, and therefore has a particular advantage when fluid overload is a problem. Excessive lipemia may be a problem in some very ill patients (eg, severe sepsis, liver failure, pancreatitis), although the clinical consequences of this are unclear. The lipid content of propofol should be taken into account in calculations of nutritional requirements when this drug is being used as a sedative.
- Appropriate water- and fat-soluble vitamin supplements should be added to the solutions.
- Although the various components of a TPN regimen can be given independently, this requires parallel adminstration of amino acid and glucose/fat solutions, which complicates administration and increases the risk of infection. As a result, many centers now use composite TPN solutions, in which all the requirements for a 24-hour period (glucose, fat, amino acids, vitamins, and trace elements, etc) are mixed aseptically in the hospital pharmacy into a single bag, volume 2–2.5 L. Drugs such as ranitidine and insulin can also be added as required.

Administration

Standard solutions are an irritant to small veins due to their high osmolarity, and therefore need to be given centrally. In the long-term convalescent patient, this should be via a single-lumen tunneled central line (usually an infraclavicular approach to the subclavian vein that has been sited under strict asepsis), which is not used for any other purpose, so as to minimize the risk of line infection. In the acute critically ill patient this is often inappropriate, but at the very least TPN solutions should be delivered via a dedicated lumen of an aseptically sited multi-lumen catheter. Solutions can be given peripherally provided that osmolarity is restricted to 900 mosmol/L, with most of the calories given in the form of lipids.

Complications
Possible complications associated with parenteral nutrition are:
- Catheter related, such as complications of insertion and residence, or sepsis (eg, entry site, bacteremia).
- Metabolic, such as hyperglycemia where insulin is often required, lipemia, hypophosphatemia which can lead to muscle weakness, reduced tissue oxygen delivery (ie, due to lack of 2,3-DPG, shifting oxyhemoglobin dissociation curve to the left), and metabolic acidosis.
- Vitamin and trace element deficiencies.
- Atrophy of the intestinal mucosal, which derives most of its nutritional requirements from the lumen of the gut rather than from the circulation. Failure to deliver nutrition enterally may therefore lead to atrophy of the intestinal mucosa and result in vascular translocation of gut bacteria.

Chapter 12

Physical injury

Brian Gehlbach
University of Chicago, Chicago, IL, USA

Trauma: basic management principles

Emergency assessment

Protocol-driven management of major trauma involves the rapid identification and treatment of life-threatening injuries (the primary survey),
followed by a systematic clinical evaluation of all injuries (the secondary
survey). Any immediate life-threatening condition, once recognized, is treated;
any deterioration requires reassessment from the beginning. Immediate
life-threatening conditions include the following:

- complete airway obstruction
- tension pneumothorax
- cardiac tamponade
- massive hemothorax.

The sequence of assessment in the primary survey is as follows:

- **A**irway and cervical spine control
- **B**reathing
- **C**irculation
- **D**ysfunction of central nervous system (CNS)
- **E**xposure.

Airway management (with protection of cervical spine)

Assume cervical spine injury if there is a history of high-speed impact, injury
of the upper torso, or head injury. Stabilize with hard collar, sandbags, and
strapping, and manage airway problems according to Figure 12.1.

Airway management

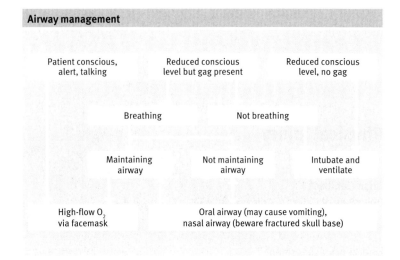

Figure 12.1 Airway management.

Breathing

For spontaneously breathing patients, administer oxygen at a concentration as high as possible; oxygen masks with a reservoir bag are suitable, being capable of delivering an inspired oxygen fraction (FiO_2) of 0.8–0.9 (80–90%). Figure 12.2 shows some of the consequences associated with inadequate ventilation and gas exchange.

Clinical assessment

This involves the usual four stages:

1. Observation – cyanosis (unreliable), external injuries, symmetry of respiratory movements, and respiratory rate and pattern
2. Palpation – tracheal and apical deviation, asymmetrical expansion, and crepitus (surgical emphysema).
3. Percussion – hyperresonance and stony dullness.
4. Auscultation.

In particular, it is important to consider the possibility of tension pneumothorax, hemothorax, and major lobar collapse.

Monitoring and investigation

Continuous arterial oxygen saturation (SaO_2) and electrocardiogram (EKG), early arterial blood gases, and chest X-ray.

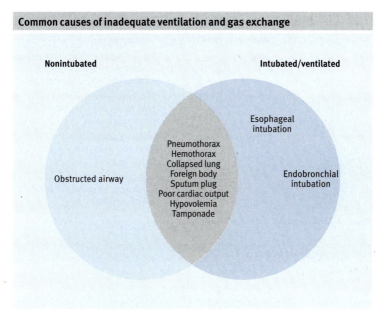

Figure 12.2 Common causes of inadequate ventilation and gas exchange.

Circulation

Clinical assessment

- peripheral circulation – poor capillary refill, cold clammy skin, core–peripheral temperature gradient
- heart rate – tachycardia, but absence does not exclude significant hypovolemia
- hypotension (Figure 12.3)
- end-organ failure – oliguria, confusion.

Monitoring

- continuous three- or five-lead EKG; full 12-lead EKG study
- regular automatic noninvasive blood pressure measurement
- urine output
- invasive arterial and central venous pressure (CVP) monitoring
- acid–base status.

Common causes of hypotension and shock in trauma

These include fractures (Figure 12.4), cardiothoracic injuries (Figure 12.5), and injuries to the abdomen, and CNS.

Hemodynamic features of blood loss

Percentage blood loss	Blood loss in 70-kg man (mL)	Clinical features
<10	<500	Postural hypotension, possibly signs of reduced peripheral perfusion, normal heart rate/blood pressure
10–20	500–1,000	Reduced peripheral perfusion, tachycardia, normal blood pressure may be maintained
20–40	1,000–2,000	Profound peripheral vasoconstriction, tachycardia, hypotension
>40	>2,000	Blood pressure becoming unrecordable, signs of end-organ failure, air hunger

Figure 12.3 Hemodynamic features of blood loss.

Blood loss caused by fractures

Pelvis	1,000–3,000 mL	Humerus	500 mL
Femur	1,000–2,000 mL	Ribs	125 mL/rib
Tibia	500–1,000 mL		

Figure 12.4 Blood loss caused by fractures.

Abdominal injuries

Severe hypovolemic shock may result from injury to intra-abdominal organs such as the spleen, liver, or kidney, or from retroperitoneal hemorrhage. Splenic injury should be suspected in a patient with left-sided subcostal or shoulder pain, particularly if there are fractures of the lower left ribs. Diagnostic peritoneal lavage (DPL) is indicated when there is hemodynamic instability with uncertain clinical findings or when a peritoneal breach is suspected following penetrating injury. Clinical criteria for a positive DPL following blunt trauma are:

- initial aspiration of >10 mL frank blood
- egress of peritoneal lavage fluid from chest drain or urinary catheter
- bile or vegetable material in lavage fluid
- red cell count >100,000/mm³ or white cell count >500/mm³
- amylase >20 IU/L.

Central nervous system injury

Hypotension must never be assumed to be due to brain or spinal cord injury until all potential causes of cardiogenic or hypovolemic shock have been excluded.

Cardiothoracic injuries

Hemothorax	Usually due to torn internal mammary or intercostal vessels
Ruptured aorta	Suspect if mediastinum is widened, particularly if associated with one or more of the following: 1. Left hemothorax 2. Depressed left main bronchus 3. Blurred outline of the aortic arch or descending aorta 4. Fractured first rib 5. Left apical hematoma 6. Right shift of the esophagus (demonstrated by nasogastric tube) Diagnosis is confirmed by arch aortography, spiral CT or transesophageal echocardiography. Immediate referral to a cardiothoracic center is required
Tension pneumothorax, cardiac tamponade, myocardialcontusions	All three present with hypotension and elevated venous pneumothorax, pressure. Clinical examination ± chest X-ray identifies cardiac pneumothorax. Tamponade may be detected by CT or echocardiography, but the clinical circumstances may require pericardial drainage on clinical grounds alone. Myocardial contusions present with heart failure, arrhythmias, and EKG abnormalities including T-wave changes and Q-waves. There may be an associated sternal fracture. Myocardial-specific cardiac isoenzymes should be measured
Penetrating cardiac injuries	Damage to any structure is possible, with predictable consequences
Concurrentmyocardial infarction	Typical EKG/enzyme changes
Systemic air embolism	More likely following penetrating chest injury; incidence unknown

Figure 12.5 Cardiothoracic injuries. CT, computed tomography; EKG, electrocardiogram.

Fluid management

At least two short, large-bore, intravenous cannulae should be sited. Patients with hypovolemic shock will require blood transfusion but, unless the patient is exsanguinating, start fluid resuscitation with 2–3 L isotonic saline given as quickly as possible while cross-matching of blood is being performed. This may be followed by colloid and cross-matched blood once it is available. The consequences of massive transfusion, notably hypothermia and coagulopathy, should be dealt with appropriately. In particular, all fluids should be warmed to avoid hypothermia. Overwhelming blood loss from the thorax, abdomen, or pelvis may require urgent/immediate operation.

The adequacy of fluid resuscitation may be monitored by urine output, which should be a minimum of 0.5 mL/kg per h, and preferably more than 1 mL/kg per h.

Dysfunction of the central nervous system

A rapid neurologic assessment can be made using either the AVPU scheme below or, if time permits, the Glasgow Coma Scale (see Chapter 6):

- **A**lert
- responds to **V**oice
- responds to **P**ain
- **U**nconscious.

Exposure

All clothing should be cut away and the patient inspected from head to toe, front and back. Warming blankets should be used.

Spinal cord injury

Two-thirds of traumatic injuries to the spine involve the cervical spine and most have associated injuries (eg, traumatic brain injury). Primary injury to the cord is a result of intrinsic trauma to the cord, external compression caused by vertebral angulation, disk protrusion, or epidural hematoma, or ischemia due to damage to the vertebral or anterior spinal arteries. The principles of management are to prevent secondary injury, which may be a consequence of one or more of the following:

- failure to maintain spinal immobility
- continued cord compression
- hypotension
- hypoxia
- cord inflammation.

Assessment of acute spinal injury

Clinical evaluation

Spinal cord injury (SCI) should be suspected in any trauma patient, particularly those presenting with neck pain or neurological features consistent with cord damage (Figure 12.6). SCI should be assumed in any patient with a depressed conscious level. Signs suggestive of cord damage in a comatose patient include:

- unexplained hypotension and bradycardia
- diaphragmatic respiratory pattern with paradoxical chest wall movement
- variable response to painful stimulation consistent with a sensory level
- reduced anal tone and priapism
- flaccid areflexia.

Spinal cord injury syndromes	
Complete neurologic injury	Total loss of sensation and motor function below level of injury. May initially be mimicked by spinal shock. Very few patients make any functional recovery if features persist for >24 h
Incomplete spinal cord injury syndromes	
Central cord syndrome	Causes: concussive cord injury with central contusion/hematoma Features: motor loss arms > legs; urinary retention; variable sensory loss below lesion
Brown–Séquard syndrome (cord hemisection)	Cause: penetrating or concussive injury to lateral aspect of the cord. Features: ipsilateral paralysis and loss of proprioception and vibration; contralateral loss of pain and temperature sensation two to three dermatomes below the lesion
Anterior cord (anterior spinal artery) syndrome	Causes: posterior protrusion of disk or bony fragment, flexion injury or disruption of anterior spinal artery Features: motor paralysis with loss of pain and temperature; sparing of posterior column modalities (propriocepion and vibration)
Posterior cord syndrome	Rare; loss of touch and proprioception

Figure 12.6 Spinal cord injury syndromes.

Radiology

Normal radiological studies do not exclude a significant spinal column injury, and a cord injury can occur without vertebral damage. Nevertheless plain spinal X-rays are the basis of radiological evaluation (Figure 12.7).

Oblique views, computed tomography (CT), and magnetic resonance imaging (MRI) studies complete the radiological evaluation. MRI provides invaluable information regarding soft tissue damage, but may be difficult to provide acutely.

Immediate field management of acute spinal injury

This is immobilization of the cervical spine in the neutral position to avoid further mechanical injury to the cord; flexion is particularly dangerous. Maintenance of airway and adequate ventilation take precedence over immobilization even if this requires jaw thrust and slight head extension.

This is followed by intravenous infusion of isotonic saline or cautious head-down positioning to improve venous return and cardiac output if the patient is hypotensive.

Early hospital management of acute spinal injury
Airway control

Tracheal intubation may be necessary for a number of reasons:

- impaired airway reflexes as a result of an associated head injury

Radiological evaluation of spinal cord injury

Radiological views of cervical spine	Features of injury
Cross-table lateral	
90% of significant cervical spine injuries are detected with this view. Since up to 14% of cervical spine injuries occur at C7, all seven cervical vertebrae must be visualized. The swimmer's modification of the lateral view may help visualize C7	1. Widening of the atlantodental interval, ie, the distance between the posterior aspect of the anterior arch of the atlas and the anterior aspect of the odontoid peg: adult >3 mm, child >5 mm 2. Loss of the lordotic alignment of the four anatomic lines of the lateral cervical spine 3. Widening of the prevertebral spaces: C3 >7 mm; C6: adult >22 mm, child >14 mm 4. Loss of intervertebral disk space: anterior narrowing = flexion injury; posterior narrowing = extension injury 5. Widening of the interspinous space. Under normal circumstances the interspinous distance remains constant or decreases from C3 downwards. An increase suggests rupture of the posterior ligaments as may occur in hyperflexion injury
Anteroposterior view	
Atlantoaxial articulation is obscured by the mandible and occiput. Demonstrates the vertical alignment of the lateral column margins, spinous, and articular processes, and depth of disk spaces. Useful in detection of unilateral facet joint injury, spinous process fractures	1. Loss of the smooth, undulating alignment of the lateral column margins 2. Abrupt deviation of a spinous process from the midline, suggestive of unilateral facet joint injury 3. Focal widening of an interspinous space, indicating hyperflexion injury
Odontoid (open-mouth) view	
Essential to evaluate relationship of C1–C2	1. Joint spaces between atlas and axis should be open and symmetrical 2. The odontoid peg should be symmetrically aligned between the lateral masses of the atlas, so that the medial atlantodental spaces are equal

Figure 12.7 Radiological evaluation of spinal cord injury.

- maxillofacial injuries
- respiratory failure as a result of high cervical cord injury, an associated severe head injury, thoracic trauma, or other major injuries
- to allow surgical treatment of spinal or other injuries.

The method chosen to intubate the trachea is determined by the skills and equipment that are available, the urgency of the need to secure the airway, the nature of the cervical injury, and the associated injuries (facial trauma, fractured base of skull, laryngeal injury). The aim is to achieve endotracheal intubation without causing further spinal injury.

If sufficient time is available, and provided that the patient is sufficiently conscious and cooperative, awake fiberoptic intubation under topical anesthesia is probably the technique of choice. If the clinical circumstances dictate rapid control of the airway, this is best achieved by direct laryngoscopy and orotracheal intubation under general anesthesia using a rapid sequence induction technique. A suggested routine in a patient with an anatomically normal airway is as follows:

- Secure good venous access and institute adequate monitoring (EKG, SaO_2, invasive blood pressure if time allows).
- Clear the airway and preoxygenate.
- The front of the rigid collar is removed and first assistant holds head in the neutral position while providing in-line stabilization of the neck.
- Administer a sleep dose of intravenous anesthetic agent followed by 1.5 mg/ kg succinylcholine (this should not be used in cord injuries that are more than 48 hours old because of the risk of life-threatening hyperkalemia). If appropriate, take steps to limit the pressor response to laryngoscopy and intubation.
- The second assistant applies cricoid pressure as the anesthetic is given.
- An experienced anesthesiologist performs laryngoscopy with a Bullard or McCoy laryngoscope.
- Reapply the rigid collar once the airway has been secured.

Emergency tracheostomy or cricothyroidotomy may be required in some critical circumstances, when the potential for secondary spinal injury becomes subordinate to life-threatening airway problems.

A suggested algorithm for airway management is shown in Figure 12.8.

Breathing

Respiratory function is often compromised in patients with cervical cord injury, for several reasons:

- mechanical ventilatory failure due to paralysis of the respiratory musculature
- poor cough, sputum retention, and atelectasis
- gastric dilation and aspiration of gastric contents
- associated airway problems arising from concurrent traumatic brain injury, maxillofacial injuries, etc
- thoracic and abdominal trauma
- neurogenic pulmonary edema.

The segmental motor innervation of the respiratory muscles is shown in Figure 12.9. The level of injury critically influences the effect on ventilation (Figure 12.10).

Airway management in acute spinal injury

Emergency		Urgent	Elective
	Uncooperative	Cooperative	Full clinical and radiological work-up
Anatomically abnormal airway	Anatomically normal airway	Awake fiberoptic intubation	Immobilize head/neck in traction device
		Failure	
Tracheostomy/ cricothyroidotomy	Rapid sequence induction In-line stabilization Direct laryngoscopy	General anesthetic + direct laryngoscopy	Awake fiberoptic or blind nasal intubation

Figure 12.8 Airway management in acute spinal injury.

Indications for ventilatory support following acute cervical spine injury can be used as objective measures of progress in nonventilated patients, and include:

- clinical features of respiratory failure
- maximum expiratory force <20 cmH_2O
- maximum inspiratory force <−20 cmH_2O
- vital capacity <15 mL/kg or <1,000 mL
- partial pressure of oxygen $(PaO_2)/FiO_2$ <250 mmHg (32.5 kPa)
- atelectasis/infiltrates on chest X-ray.

Patients with lesions above C5 (unable to move hands or arms) usually require ventilation. Patients with intact C5 innervation (can shrug shoulders and externally rotate arms) may maintain adequate respiratory function in the absence of any other pulmonary insult. Patients with lesions at C6 will usually manage without ventilatory support in the acute phase. Tracheostomy should be considered in patients likely to require ventilatory support for more than 2 weeks.

Management of the spontaneously breathing patient with acute spinal cord injury includes the following:

- close observation – respiratory failure requiring mechanical ventilation may develop in the days following injury, and results from sputum retention, gastric dilation, and diaphragmatic splinting, progression of other

Innervation of the respiratory muscles

Inspiratory		Expiratory	
Infrahyoid	C1–3	Erector spinae	C1–S5
Sternomastoid	C1–3	Trapezius	C1–4
Trapezius	C1–4	Serratus anterior	C5–7
Levator scapulae	C3–5	Latissimus dorsi	C6–8
Diaphragm	C3–5	Intercostals	T1–11
Scalenes	C4–8	Transversus abdominis	T6–L1
Pectorals	C5–T1	Rectus abdominis	T6–12
Serratus anterior	C5–7	Internal oblique	T6–L1
Intercostals	T1–11	Serratus posterior inferior	T9–12
Costal levators	T1–11		
Serratus posterior superior	T2–5		

Figure 12.9 Innervation of the respiratory muscles. Primary respiratory muscles are shown in blue and accessory muscles are in normal type.

injuries, etc. Serial measurement of vital capacity etc, may help to objectively follow progress

- nursing in the supine position: respiratory function deteriorates in the sitting position
- humidified controlled oxygen therapy
- intensive chest physiotherapy – specialist centers use techniques such as nasal suction, regular deep breathing exercises, incentive spirometry, and assisted coughing
- careful fluid balance
- adequate (enteral) nutrition.

Circulation

The initial response to acute cervical cord injury is a brief sympathetic storm, leading to severe systemic and pulmonary hypertension, myocardial dysfunction, and occasionally neurogenic pulmonary edema. This is followed by a period of spinal shock that may last for some weeks. The cardiovascular consequences of profound loss of sympathetic tone include the following:

- Reduction in peripheral vascular resistance and subsequent hypotension.
- Sinus bradycardia due to unopposed vagal tone.
- Dilation of venous capacitance vessels leading to venous pooling, reduced venous filling pressures, and a relative hypovolemia.

Acute spinal injury and ventilation

Level of injury	Effect on respiratory function	Clinical features
Above C3	Paralysis of all primary muscles of inspiration and expiration (diaphragm, intercostals, and abdominals)	Immediate respiratory failure; intubation and ventilation required
C3–5	Paralysis of all primary expiratory muscles (intercostals, abdominals); variable loss of diaphragmatic function depending upon level of injury; FRC is reduced to 20–25% normal; FVC <1 L; expiratory flow <2 L/s; increased residual volume	Paradoxical ventilation (ie, chest wall retraction during inspiration, expansion during expiration); respiratory function improves in supine position; no cough; increased use of upper accessory muscles (sternomastoid, etc); ventilatory support may be required, and mandatory for lesions above C4
C5–8	Paralysis of all primary expiratory muscles (intercostals, abdominals); loss of intercostal activity also interferes with the normal function of the diaphragm even though its innervation is preserved; FRC is reduced to 30% normal, with similar reductions in FVC and expiratory flow rates	As for C3–5 lesions; respiratory function may be adequate initially, but deterioration in subsequent days can be anticipated
T1–6	Variable loss of intercostal function; efficiency of diaphragm reduced	Weak cough
T7–12	Reduced abdominal muscle activity	Weak cough

Figure 12.10 Acute spinal injury and ventilation. FRC, functional residual capacity; FVC, forced vital capacity.

- Risk of profound bradycardia or even asystole in response airway instrumentation.
- Inability to mount appropriate response to hypovolemia.

Spinal shock is a diagnosis of exclusion; hypovolemia in particular must be ruled out. In the acute period, hypotension may contribute to secondary cord injury and should therefore be treated aggressively. A mean arterial pressure of 80–90 mmHg should be maintained, and some advocate inducing a hyperdynamic state with careful hypervolemia and, if necessary, inotropic support, as guided by invasive monitoring. The choice of inotrope depends upon the intrinsic heart rate and resting vascular tone. Pre-treatment with atropine may be necessary if reactive bradycardias are troublesome.

Neurosurgical management

All possible measures to minimize further neck movement should be employed. Initial immobilization (Figure 12.11) should be with a rigid collar, lateral sandbags, and forehead taping, which should be maintained during all preliminary assessment and resuscitation. Secondary stabilization with tong/halo traction depends upon the nature of the injury and the practice of the particular neurosurgical unit, as does the decision for any surgical intervention.

The effectiveness of pharmacologic treatment of secondary cord injury remains uncertain. Some centers recommend methylprednisolone 30 mg/kg as a slow bolus, followed by 5.4 mg/kg per h for 23 hours by continuous infusion, started as soon as possible after injury.

Effectiveness of various immobilization techniques

Immobilization technique	Motion still permitted
Soft collar	96% flexion, 73% extension, 100% rotation
Rigid collar	30% extension/flexion, 45% rotation
Lateral sandbags and forehead tape	No flexion; 35% extension, 5% rotation
Tong/halo traction	4% flexion/extension, 1% rotation

Figure 12.11 Effectiveness of various immobilization techniques.

Chronic post-transection period

The acute post-transection phase of flaccid paralysis and spinal shock is gradually replaced in the ensuing weeks with long-term spastic paralysis (Figure 12.12). Such changes in the respiratory musculature are associated with improvement in respiratory function, vital capacity, etc, and may be the time when ventilatory support can be weaned. Other problems include:

- Autonomic hyperreflexia – a proportion of patients with lesions above T7 will exhibit exaggerated autonomic and motor responses to triggers such as bladder and bowel distension, movement, etc. They are characterized by hypertension, bradycardia, and vasodilation above the spinal level of injury (both reflex responses to the hypertension), sweating, and hypertonicity. Treatment includes α blockade and meticulous bladder and bowel care.
- Spastic paralysis – although the onset of spasticity improves respiratory function, it creates problems with general care, posture, and positioning. Aggressive physiotherapy is required to prevent fixed contractures.
- Depression.

Other systemic problems in acute cord injury

System	Problems	Management
Gastrointestinal	Loss of sympathetic tone, leading to gastric dilation, gastric stasis, paralytic ileus, intestinal dilation	Nasogastric tube, enteral feeding when gastrointestinal function returns, laxatives, enemas, manual evacuation
	Stress ulceration	Gastric mucosal prophylaxis with sucralfate or H_2-receptor antagonists
Genitourinary	Bladder distension Urinary retention Chronic infection	Indwelling urinary catheter initially, intermittent catheterization later High risk of infection, which must be distinguished from colonization
Integument	Pressure sores	Clinical attention to pressure areas, pressure-relieving mattresses, good nutrition
Metabolic	Poikilothermia in lesions below T1, leading to hypothermia Malnutrition due to intestinal stasis Metabolic alkalosis due to excessive gastric acid aspiration, possibly resulting in respiratory compensation and hypoventilation Life-threatening hyperkalemic response to succinylcholine if used after 48 h; danger persists for up to a year	Recognition and heat-preserving measures. Enteral nutrition if possible; parenteral nutrition may be necessary

Figure 12.12 Other systemic problems in acute cord injury.

Electrical injury

Introduction

The current (I) flowing through a conductor of resistance Ω is determined by the potential difference V across the conductor thus:

$$I = V/\Omega$$

with the energy dissipated as heat by the current flow being given by:

$$\text{Power} = V \times I = I^2\Omega$$

For current to flow through the body, an electrical circuit must be completed; this usually entails passage of the current to earth, the path taken through the body being determined by the site of entry and the site of contact with earth. The consequences of current flow through biological tissue depend upon the following:

- The magnitude of the current flow, which in turn is determined by the potential difference applied and the resistance of the tissue. The principal electrical resistance of the body is provided by (dry) skin (skin > bone > muscle > nerves > blood vessels), although this falls from >100,000 Ω to 1,000 Ω when the skin is wet. It follows that, if the domestic electrical supply of 120 V is applied to the skin, the current flow will be 120 mA if the skin is wet in comparison to 0.124 mA if dry.
- The time for which the current is applied.
- The nature and volume of the tissue(s) through which the current passes, which in turn are determined by the path to earth and the relative electrical conductivities of the tissues involved. For instance, if a current is applied to a finger it will flow preferentially through the soft tissues rather than bone, since the former have a much higher conductivity. As the volume of such tissue is low in a finger, the heating effect will be marked and thermal injury is likely. In contrast, the soft tissue of the forearm is more extensive and the heating effect is therefore much reduced.

Types of electrical injury

A macroshock injury is one that follows the passage of an electric current through the body surface to internal organs (notably the heart). High-tension injuries are when static electricity builds up on an insulator until such time as it discharges to earth, in so doing heating the air through which it passes and thereby generating a spark. Microshock injuries include a myocardial injury that follows the delivery of an electrical current directly into the heart. These are all discussed in more detail below.

Macroshock
Thermal injury
Currents in excess of 1 A generate sufficient heat to inflict a thermal injury on the tissues through which they pass. As noted above, this effect is maximized when the current passes through a small volume of tissue.

Myocardium
Currents in the region of 100 mA are capable of causing life-threatening electrical dysfunction of the heart by inducing ventricular fibrillation.

Larger currents cause mechanical disruption of the heart tissue, resulting in myocardial dysfunction that lasts for some days and that can be associated with EKG changes and elevated cardiac-specific muscle enzymes.

Skeletal muscle

Although currents of 10 mA are not directly damaging in themselves, the tetanic contractions that they induce cause the 'no let go' phenomenon and thereby prolong exposure to the harmful insult. Larger currents cause direct thermal injury to muscles and their vasculature. The resulting myoglobinuria may lead to acute renal failure.

Vascular tissue

Blood vessels are particularly sensitive to thermal injury from electric currents, with the resulting destructive thrombotic process causing distal ischemia.

Nervous tissue

Both peripheral and central nervous tissue injury may occur. Spinal cord damage presents with paraplegia, while intracranial electrical injury can cause coma and central apnea.

High-tension injuries

Voltages in excess of 1,000 V are involved and are generally derived from industrial electrical sources or lightning strikes (Figure 12.13). The following are the presenting features:

- Extensive thermal injury that results from the high currents involved.
- Mechanical injuries that are a consequence of the violent muscular contractions induced by the shock; fractures, joint dislocations, and extensive muscle injury can result.
- Coma and brain-stem areflexia (potentially reversible despite initial features).

Management involves ensuring that the environment is safe for rescuers, and cardiopulmonary resuscitation. Specific therapies for particular injuries include:

- cardiorespiratory support
- arteriography to define integrity of blood supply to a tissue
- débridement/excision of necrotic tissue; fasciotomies may be required
- management of orthopedic injuries when appropriate
- mannitol if there is a risk of myoglobinuria and renal failure.

Consequences of electrical macroshock	
Current	Effect
300–500 μA	Tingling
>1 mA	Painful
10–15 mA	Tetanic muscle contraction, leading to the 'no let go' phenomenon
50 mA	Tetanic paralysis of the respiratory muscles; slow death by asphyxia ('blue asphyxia')
75–100 mA	Ventricular fibrillation
1 A	Tissue injury and burns
5 A	Asystole (defibrillator principle)

Figure 12.13 Consequences of electrical macroshock.

Microshock

A current as low as 50 mA can induce fatal ventricular fibrillation when it is delivered directly into a chamber of the heart, as opposed to delivery across the heart from body surface to surface, when the effects would be trivial. The requirements for such microshock are an intravascular device that can conduct the current into the heart, such as a central line, pulmonary artery catheter, or temporary pacing device. In addition to this, a source for such a current (eg, a patient monitor with sufficient leakage current) is also required. It may be connected to the intravascular device directly, or the connection may be made by an attendant who touches the device and a piece of electrical equipment simultaneously (the current being too small for the attendant to notice). Prevention of microshock is as follows:

- Use electrical equipment with a leakage current of <10 mA.
- Electrical isolation of the patient: earthing of the patient must be avoided if possible.
- Patient handling: avoid touching the patient and electrical equipment simultaneously.

Burns

Pathophysiology

A severe thermal injury has both local and systemic consequences; eg, life-threatening airway obstruction may rapidly follow upper airway burns, and edema of circumferential burns to the torso or limbs can, by a tourniquet effect, cause respiratory embarrassment and limb ischemia, respectively. The immediate systemic consequences of a severe burn result largely from the massive fluid and electrolyte losses from the burn, which in turn lead to so-called 'burns shock'. Finally, an established severe thermal injury evokes a systemic inflammatory reaction indistinguishable from sepsis, which is characterized by a hyperdynamic, hypercatabolic state that can progress to multiple organ dysfunction and death. Figure 12.14 shows the pathophysiologic consequences associated with a severe burn.

Assessment of the size of the burn
The severity of a burn injury is determined by the depth of the burn (Figure 12.15) and its extent, and also by anatomic location. Second- and third-degree burns in excess of 15–20% in an adult, or 10–15% in a child, require intravenous fluid resuscitation. An extensive smoke inhalation or thermal injury of the respiratory tract is equivalent to up to 30% full-thickness burn. A rapid estimate of percentage burn size upon which to base initial fluid resuscitation can be made using the rule of nines (excluding areas of simple erythema), which indicates the percentage of body area accounted for by different body parts:

- head and arms 9% each
- legs 18% each
- front and back of trunk 18% each.

This method tends to overestimate the extent of the burn. Burn extent is more accurately assessed using the Lund and Browder chart (Figures 12.16 and 12.17), which takes into account the effect of age on body proportions.

Management
Respiratory care
The airway may be compromised because of associated head trauma, cerebral hypoxemia, or upper airway burns. The management of smoke inhalation and upper airway burns is described later; in general it is safer to intubate the airway early. Supplemental oxygen therapy should be given, and monitored with arterial blood gas analysis and pulse oximetry. A carboxyhemoglobin level should be obtained to exclude carbon monoxide poisoning. The need for ventilatory support should be assessed in the usual fashion.

Circulation
Intravenous fluid resuscitation is required in significant burns (adults >15%, children >10%, less if there is associated smoke inhalation injury). In most regimens, the hourly fluid requirement is calculated from the extent of the burn and time after injury, fluid requirements being greatest in the first 12 hours. The Parkland formula is commonly used to calculate fluid requirements. There is no agreement on which fluids should be used, and in

Pathophysiologic consequences of a severe burn

Cardiovascular	A severe thermal injury leads to massive losses of plasma and water from the intravascular space, and to life-threatening hypovolemic shock. Such fluid losses occur not only in burn tissue but also in normal tissues if the burn exceeds 20% of body surface area. A patient with a 50% burn can lose a third of the total blood volume within 3–4 h, with the hematocrit rising to 60–70%. Myocardial depression induced by the emerging inflammatory response may add to the shock state Hemolytic anemia – 1% red cell mass/1% burn Dilutional and disseminated intravascular coagulopathies Thrombocytopenia
Gastrointestinal	High incidence of stress ulceration
Metabolic	Massive stress response, characterized by: (a) a hyperdynamic state associated with increased O_2 requirements and CO_2 production (b) increased plasma catecholamines, cortisol, and other stress hormones; cortisol levels may be $10 \times$ normal, and are maximal on day 2 (c) hypercatabolic state, with glucose intolerance, and increased gluconeogenesis from muscle and fat breakdown; muscle wasting and nutritional failure are common (d) increased antidiuretic hormone secretion resulting in water retention and possible hyponatremia The hypermetabolic state described above is amplified by: (a) pain, requiring adequate analgesia (b) sepsis, requiring effective identification and treatment of infection (c) heat loss: evaporative losses from exposed tissues results in heat loss, the response to which is to increase heat production by increasing metabolism; this process can be attenuated by increasing the environmental temperature to 25–33°C and by effecting prompt coverage with skin grafts, etc Increased susceptibility to infection
Renal	Prerenal oliguric renal failure resulting from hypovolemic shock Acute tubular necrosis resulting from: (a) myoglobinuria (extensive muscle injury) (b) hemoglobinuria (intravascular hemolysis) (c) SIRS (d) sepsis
Respiratory	Smoke inhalational injury to lower respiratory tract Thermal injury to upper airway, resulting in edema and obstruction, the onset of which may be rapid. Maximal edema formation occurs at 24 h, subsiding after 4 days Tourniquet effect of circumferential full-thickness burns around the thorax leading to restrictive lung defect Acute lung injury and ARDS, the pulmonary manifestation of the systemic inflammatory response to severe burns The hypermetabolic consequences of a severe burn injury results in increased CO_2 production Bronchopneumonia

Figure 12.14 Pathophysiologic consequences of a severe burn. ARDS, acute respiratory distress syndrome; SIRS, systemic inflammatory response syndrome.

Classification of burn depth

Classification	Features
First degree (superficial, partial)	Limited to epithelial layer of the skin Very painful and erythematous Excluded from estimates of percentage burn Heals well
Second degree (deep, partial)	Extends to dermis Painful Heals more slowly
Third degree (full thickness)	Analgesic Full-thickness burn tissue is unable to stretch in response to underlying edema, and circumferential full-thickness burns thereby exert a tourniquet effect that may compromise tissue perfusion and require urgent release or 'escharotomy'

Figure 12.15 Classification of burn depth.

particular there is controversy on the relative roles of crystalloid versus colloid solutions. The priority is the recognition of the fluid requirement rather than the type of fluid and the essential ingredients are salt (Na^+ 130–150 mmol/L) and water. Specific problems with fluid therapy include:

- hypovolemia and shock
- fluid overload and peripheral/airway/pulmonary edema
- dilutional coagulopathy
- electrolyte imbalance
- hyponatremia
- hypernatremia
- hyperkalemia
- hypocalcemia
- the development of the systemic inflammatory response syndrome (SIRS), with consequent systemic peripheral and pulmonary edema, often necessitating invasive monitoring and inotropic support
- evaporative water losses from uncovered burns, leading to hypernatremia
- renal failure.

Some centers use regimens that include colloid as 4.5% human albumin solution (HAS), blood, and crystalloid (administered according to the schedule in Figure 12.18), although the use of albumin solution in the critically ill is controversial and has not been shown to improve survival. The adequacy of fluid resuscitation should be judged by the following:

- clinical assessment – capillary return, venous filling, core–peripheral temperature gradient, urine output: adults: 0.5–1 mL/kg per h; children: 1–2 mL/kg per h

Lund and Browder chart

	Age (years)					
	<1	1	5	10	15	Adult
A = ½ head (%)	9.5	8.5	6.5	5.5	4.25	3.5
B = ½ thigh (%)	2.75	3.25	4	4.25	4.5	4.75
C = ½ leg (%)	2.5	2.5	2.75	3	3.25	3.5

Figure 12.16 Lund and Browder chart.

Lund and Browder chart

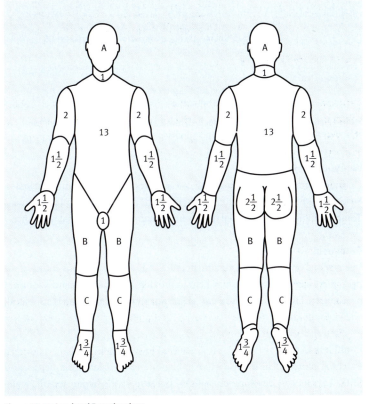

Figure 12.17 Lund and Browder chart.

- serial hematocrit estimations – man (45%), woman (40%) child (35%)
- urine osmolality
- CVP monitoring in difficult cases.

Administration schedule for HAS, blood, and crystalloid

Fluid	Administration
HAS (4.5%)	1. Divide the first 48 h into seven periods of 4 h, 4 h, 4 h, 6 h, 6 h, 12 h, 12 h 2. Give 0.5 mL/kg for each percentage of BSA during the first 4-h period (catching up for lost time) 3. At the end of this period assess the volume status of the patient (see below). If resuscitation is judged to be correct continue with the same volumes in subsequent periods; if not adjust appropriately 4. Plasma deficit can be estimated from measured Hct: Deficit = BV − (BV × predicted Hct/measured Hct)
Blood (as packed cells)	1. 10–25% burns: 1% blood volume for each percentage BSA involved in sixth period only 2. >25% burns: 1% blood volume for each percentage BSA involved in second and sixth periods
Crystalloid (as 5% dextrose or oral fluids)	1. In uncovered burns water losses can be considerable; give 2 L per 10% burn per 24 h 2. If wounds are dressed give 1.5–2 mL/kg per h 3. Reduce if hyponatremia begins to develop

Figure 12.18 Administration schedule for HAS, blood, and crystalloid. BSA, body surface area; BV, estimated blood volume; HAS, human albumin solution; Hct, hematocrit.

Wound management

Débridement and resurfacing within 24–36 hours reduces fluid and heat losses. Strict asepsis is mandatory; topical chemotherapy may reduce infection rates. Topical antibiotics are avoided due to risk of subsequent bacterial resistance.

Analgesia

Intravenous opioids can be administered as a bolus, continuous infusion, or patient controlled. Entonox may help to provide additional analgesia for brief procedures. Figure 12.18 shows an administration schedule for HAS, blood, and crystalloid.

Renal impairment

Potential causes include hypovolemia, hemo- and myoglobinuria, sepsis, and SIRS. Uremia can develop very quickly because of the hypercatabolic state. Mannitol 1 g/kg is advocated in cases of hemo- and myoglobinuria, but care should be taken not to precipitate pulmonary edema.

Nutritional support

As noted above, a significant burn injury initiates a marked hypermetabolic stress response. This mandates a corresponding increase in calorie and protein intake to minimize fat and protein catabolism and muscle wasting. Wherever possible, nutrition should be delivered enterally to preserve intestinal mucosal integrity, and thereby minimize bacterial translocation. A variety of formulae for calculating requirements are available, for example:

$$\text{Calories (given as carbohydrate + fat)} = 20 \text{ kcal/kg body weight} + 70 \text{ kcal/\% burn}$$

$$\text{Protein} = 1 \text{ g/kg body weight} + 3 \text{ g/\% burn}$$

Glucose intolerance is common, and insulin may be required. Iron and vitamin supplementation is also advised. Some advocate the use of feeds rich in glutamine and omega-3 fatty acids in order to improve immune function.

Prognosis
Factors influencing outcome include depth and extent of burn, inhalational injury, renal impairment, age, and chronic health status. As a rough guide:

$$\text{\% mortality} = \text{\% area burn} + \text{age (years)}$$

Smoke inhalation
The consequences of a smoke inhalation injury are thermal injury, which is largely restricted to the upper airway due to reflex closure of the glottis and dissipation of the thermal energy by the airways. It results in edema of the upper airway and large bronchi. Complete upper airway obstruction may develop rapidly. Distal pulmonary damage, resulting from the inhalation of toxic and corrosive chemicals such as hydrochloric acid, phosgene, oxides of sulfur, and nitrogen, may also occur. This results in bronchiolitis, alveolitis, and respiratory failure. The fluid losses associated with such pulmonary edema may contribute to 'burn shock' syndrome. Inhalation of the toxic products of combustion such as carbon monoxide and cyanide may also occur.

Clinical features
The following clinical features suggest an inhalational injury:
- fire within an enclosed space
- burns/soot around face, neck, or mouth
- carbonaceous sputum
- stridor, hoarseness, wheeze or respiratory difficulty
- altered conscious level.

The chest X-ray may be normal in the acute period, and therefore often unhelpful.

Management

Thermal injury to the airways

Life-threatening airway obstruction can progress very rapidly, but the onset may be delayed for up to 24 hours following injury, and should be treated by immediate intubation. Anyone suspected of suffering inhalational injury should be continuously monitored in a high-dependency environment in which impending airway problems can be promptly identified. Indications for intubation include:

- stridor or dysphonia
- hypoxemia or hypercapnia
- facial burns with depressed conscious level
- facial burns plus circumferential neck burns
- full-thickness burns to nose and lips
- pharyngeal edema.

It should be emphasized that there is no place for conservative management in such circumstances; it is better to intubate unnecessarily than to delay and be presented with complete obstruction. The method of tracheal intubation depends upon the clinical circumstances.

Awake fiberoptic intubation with topical analgesia is attractive, but may be difficult in a distressed, hypoxic patient. Cautious laryngoscopy following an inhalational induction may be preferred, but again may be difficult. Intravenous induction may result in complete airway obstruction. Endotracheal intubation is likely to be impossible if there is complete airway obstruction, and the appropriate personnel and facilities must be available to proceed immediately to an emergency tracheostomy, a procedure that may be difficult in the presence of cervical burns. Whatever technique is employed, it must be carried out by an experienced anesthesiologist. Once the airway is intubated, the extent of the thermal injury to the lower respiratory tract should be defined by fiberoptic bronchoscopy, which may reveal carbonaceous sputum, mucosal ulceration, bleeding, or edema. Inspired gas should be humidified and bronchospasm treated in the usual fashion. Airway edema is usually maximal 24 hours post-burn, and resolves after 4–5 days. Steroids are not recommended because of the risk of infection.

Distal pulmonary damage and respiratory failure

Respiratory failure and the need for mechanical ventilation should be assessed and managed in the usual fashion (as noted below, carbon monoxide poisoning complicates the assessment of oxygenation). Defects in gas exchange may be severe, particularly if acute respiratory distress syndrome

(ARDS) develops, and a lung protective strategy utilizing low tidal ventilation should be instituted.

Carbon monoxide poisoning

Carbon monoxide (CO) interferes with tissue oxygenation in several ways: it binds avidly to hemoglobin (the affinity of CO for hemoglobin is 250 times that of O_2), and thereby prevents oxygen carriage; it promotes a left shift of the oxyhemoglobin dissociation curve, making hemoglobin less likely to give up oxygen to the tissues; and it binds to other heme proteins such as the cytochrome oxidases, and so impairs oxidative processes at the mitochondrial level. It is this, rather than binding to hemoglobin (Hb), that is principally responsible for the toxic effects of CO.

The clinical features of CO poisoning include nausea and vomiting, headache, hyperventilation, hypotension, increased muscle tone, and coma. Classically patients appear with cherry-pink skin, although cyanosis is more common. Pulse oximeters over-read because they are unable to distinguish carboxy-hemoglobin (HbCO) from oxyhemoglobin (HbO_2). Arterial blood gases and spectroscopic analysis of the blood reveals the true picture of a normal partial pressure of oxygen (PaO_2), a low arterial oxygen saturation (SaO_2), and a high HbCO level. While blood spectroscopy can be performed manually by the hematology service, many blood gas analyzers now have a co-oximetry facility that measures blood HbO_2 and HbCO levels in seconds, although beware of older analyzers that calculate the oxygen saturation from the measured PaO_2. HbCO levels of 20% suggest a significant inhalation injury, while levels of 60% are life threatening.

Treatment is largely supportive, specific measures including oxygen therapy. Treatment with high inspired oxygen concentrations promotes the displacement of CO from heme-binding sites. The relationship between the half-life of HbCO and inspired oxygen concentration is shown in Figure 12.19.

Oxygen should be delivered at the highest concentration available by face-mask (a mask with reservoir bag, or by high-flow circuit) or by intubation and ventilation with 100% oxygen as appropriate. Clearance from tissue-binding sites is slower than from hemoglobin, and therapy is therefore maintained until the systemic consequences of poisoning (acidosis, coma, etc) resolve, rather than according to HbCO concentrations.

Hyperbaric oxygen therapy (1–2 hours at 3 atmospheres, repeated after 24 hours) is more effective than normobaric oxygen therapy, and reduces long-term neurologica sequelae. Although its limited access restricts its usefulness

Oxygen concentration and half-life of HbCO	
Oxygen concentration	Half-life of HbCO (min)
Air	240
100% oxygen, 1 atmosphere	60
100% oxygen, 3 atmospheres	23

Figure 12.19 **Oxygen concentration and half-life of HbCO.** HbCO, carboxyhemoglobin.

somewhat, transfer to the nearest hyperbaric chamber should be considered in the following circumstances:

- failure to respond to conventional therapy
- coma (regardless of HbCO levels)
- HbCO levels >40%
- pregnancy.

Cyanide poisoning

Combustion of synthetic fabrics and furnishings generates cyanide and other toxic products. Any patient with evidence of inhalational injury should be treated for cyanide poisoning with 10 mL 3% sodium nitrite over 3 minutes followed by 25 mL 50% sodium thiosulphate over 10 minutes.

Prognosis

A significant thermal injury to the respiratory tract worsens the prognosis in the burns patient, with a proportion developing ARDS.

Near drowning

Drowning is, unfortunately, a common cause of death in children. In adults, it is commonly associated with drug and alcohol abuse. The consequences of near drowning are shown in Figure 12.20. Near drowning is the clinical syndrome that develops in individuals who survive an immersion episode.

Pathophysiology

The immediate consequences of immersion are shown in Figure 12.21. Initially, immersion induces a voluntary breath-holding period along with the so-called 'diving reflex'. This apnea eventually breaks under the intense stimulation of a rising partial pressure of carbon dioxide ($PaCO_2$), with subsequent inspiration leading to the inhalation of the immersion fluid. The consequences thereafter depend upon whether reflex laryngospasm prevents significant aspiration ('dry drowning').

Consequences of near drowning

Cardiovascular	EKG may be abnormal; hemodynamic performance may be impaired by hypoxia and acidosis, hypothermia, pulmonary and systemic vasoconstriction, and fluid losses into the lungs (particularly if the alveolar–capillary barrier is disrupted). Intravascular hemolysis is rarely a problem
Metabolic	Hypothermia may complicate resuscitation, but may also aid survival and neurologic recovery. Inhalation of a volume of fluid sufficient to disturb ionic homeostasis is very uncommon in survivors
Neurologic	Initial neurologic assessment may be complicated by hypothermia, drug and alcohol abuse, head injury, seizures, etc. Cerebral edema may develop in response to cerebral ischemia
Respiratory	Inhalation of as little as 2.5 mL/kg can cause marked pulmonary insufficiency, features including increased airway resistance, loss of surfactant, alveolar flooding with disruption of the alveolar–capillary barrier, reduced lung compliance, intense pulmonary vasoconstriction, and severe hypoxemia. ARDS may develop, occasionally after an intervening period of recovery

Figure 12.20 Consequences of near drowning. ARDS, acute respiratory distress syndrome; EKG, electrocardiogram.

Clinical features

The features of near drowning include the pathophysiologic consequences of the immersion, the nature of the drowning episode, hypothermia, and associated problems (eg, drug abuse, cervical spine, and head trauma).

Investigations

These include:

- arterial blood gases
- urea and electrolytes
- complete blood count, clotting studies
- urine/plasma for free hemoglobin, serum haptoglobin
- EKG
- chest X-ray
- head CT and cervical spine studies as indicated.

Management

Initial measures

Continue initial life-support measures until details of the immersion episode are established. Resuscitation measures should not be abandoned prematurely in young hypothermic patients who have suffered cold-water drowning.

Consequences of immersion

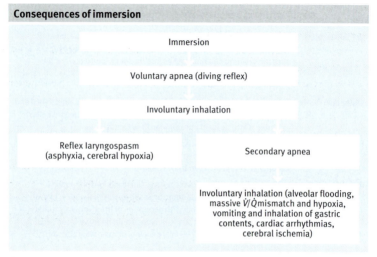

Figure 12.21 Consequences of immersion.

Airway and breathing

Lung drainage procedures are of dubious value. Intubation and ventilation are usually required, with maneuvers such as the positive end-expiratory pressure (PEEP), inverse-ratio ventilation, employed to deal with severe oxygenation defects of acute lung injury.

Circulation

Circulatory support should be undertaken with fluids and inotropes as directed by invasive monitoring.

Neurologic

Maintenance of cerebral perfusion, oxygenation, and normocapnia is a sensible measure in patients who have suffered a significant cerebral ischemic episode. A head CT scan may demonstrate cerebral edema and also exclude focal pathology. Intracranial pressure monitoring is controversial, but may be indicated in severe cases. Intracranial hypertension is treated as directed elsewhere. Moderate hypothermia may afford some cerebral protection, but there is no place for barbiturate coma.

Other measures

Insert a nasogastric tube to decompress the stomach, which may be distended with swallowed fluid. Rewarm gently, but avoid hyperthermia.

Outcome

There are several factors that may influence recovery:

- Age: younger victims (particularly children) have more potential for good neurological recovery.
- Type of drowning: cold immersion and 'dry drowning' have better outcomes.
- Volume of aspirate: >22 mL/kg invariably fatal.
- Duration of submersion: >10 minutes associated with poor outcome.

Cardiopulmonary resuscitation (CPR) that lasts more than 25 minutes, fixed and dilated pupils, a pH that is less than 7.0, and absent/abnormal movements 24 hours after injury are all features that predict poor recovery. Despite these factors that may influence recovery, resuscitation and treatment should not be abandoned early, especially in young children following cold-water immersion.

Hypothermia

Hypothermia often goes unrecognized, and is more common in children because they have a large surface area to body weight ratio and in elderly people because of impaired thermoregulation/shivering. Hypothermia is defined as a core temperature of 35°C or less, and can be arbitrarily subdivided as shown in Figure 12.22. It can be induced as part of a clinical maneuver (eg, cardiopulmonary bypass, treatment of head injury), or it can be accidental. Accidental hypothermia is more likely to be severe if thermoregulation is impaired; eg, in elderly people or in individuals with untreated hypothyroidism. Figure 12.23 summarizes the pathophysiology of hypothermia.

Diagnosis

A high index of suspicion is necessary in many cases, and a suitable low-reading thermometer may be required. Rectal temperature, commonly used in unconscious patients, may be up to 0.5°C higher than core temperature, and changes here lag behind if deep body temperature is changing rapidly. Other measures of

Classification of hypothermia by temperature	
Type	Core temperature (°C)
Mild	32–35
Moderate	28–32
Severe	20–28
Profound	<20

Figure 12.22 Classification of hypothermia by temperature.

Pathophysiology of hypothermia

System	Physiologic effects of cold
Cardiovascular	
Mild hypothermia	Sympathetic stimulation, resulting in tachycardia, peripheral vasoconstriction, and increased cardiac output (associated with shivering)
Moderate/ severe hypothermia	Progressive slowing of cardiac conduction leads to bradycardia, widening of PR, QRS, and QT intervals, and emergence of 'J' waves (extra deflection between QRS and T-waves) at temperatures below 33°C. Myocardial irritability (trivial insults such as moving a patient may precipitate tachyrrhythmias). Atrial fibrillation is common between 28 and 35°C, and ventricular fibrillation may occur below 28°C. Direct depression of myocardial contractility with falling core temperature, so that the cardiac output becomes insufficient to meet metabolic demands. Hypovolemia and hemoconcentration due to excessive renal losses
Extremities	Brief local cooling below 12°C of limbs (eg, immersion injury) induces a reversible motor and sensory paralysis. If cold immersion persists for some hours then permanent injury to nervous and muscular tissue becomes more likely. Frostbite is the freezing of tissue extremities; loss of both frozen and underlying nonfrozen tissue can be anticipated
Metabolic	Basal metabolic rate is high in the shivering phase but declines at a rate of 5–7% per °C cooling. A metabolic acidosis is common, and results from an accumulation of lactate and failure of H^+ secretion by the kidney. It partially counteracts the hypothermia-induced left shift in the oxyhemoglobin dissociation curve. Failure of glucose utilization and hyperglycemia. Hyperkalemia due to failure of the Na^+/K^+ membrane pumps. Hypoxic liver damage
Neurologic	Stepwise reduction in cerebral activity: 1. <35°C: confusion, amnesia, reduced conscious level 2. <30°C: unconsciousness and pupillary dilation 3. <20°C: flat EEG Matched reduction in cerebral blood flow and cerebral metabolic rate. (Brain) death cannot be diagnosed if core temperature <35°C
Renal	With mild hypothermia sympathetic activity leads to an increase in the central blood volume, which in turn promotes a diuresis ('cold' diuresis). Renal blood flow and glomerular filtration fall with progressive hypothermia. Salt and water losses may persist due to metabolic failure of renal tubules
Respiratory	Minute ventilation changes according to metabolic demands, an increase with shivering being followed by a progressive fall as metabolism slows. Reduced oxygen tissue delivery due to left shift of the oxyhemoglobin dissociation curve. Impaired hypoxic pulmonary vasoconstriction. Impaired cough reflex, with increased risk of aspiration
Others	Reduced gastrointestinal motility and ileus. Muscular rigidity below 33°C. Leukopenia and immunosuppression. Thrombocytopenia, coagulopathy, and disseminated intravascular coagulation. Pancreatitis. Thawing of tissues suffering severe frostbite can result in a syndrome resembling crush injury, in which life-threatening hyperkalemia and acidosis can develop

Figure 12.23 Pathophysiology of hypothermia. EEG, electroencephalogram; K^+, potassium; Na^+, sodium.

core temperature include flowing urine, the tympanic membrane, and esophageal and blood temperature (from pulmonary artery catheter).

Management
Airway and breathing
Patients in a coma or respiratory failure should be intubated and ventilated. Inspired gases should be warmed and humidified.

Circulation
In cases of cardiac arrest, advanced life support should be continued until the core temperature is at least 32–35°C. In severe hypothermia, cardiac massage can precipitate ventricular fibrillation, and it has therefore been suggested that, even if peripheral pulses are absent, chest compression should be avoided if the EKG shows sinus rhythm and the core temperature is less than 28°C. The 2005 American Heart Association guidelines for emergency cardiovascular care address the specific management of perfusing and nonperfusing rhythms in various states of hypothermia.

Establish secure venous access, if possible by the central venous route. This not only guides fluid resuscitation and allows the administration of vasoactive drugs, but also may be technically easier than peripheral access in patients who are intensely vasoconstricted. Resuscitate with 0.9% saline with 5% glucose, and warm all intravenous fluids.

Inotropes may precipitate ventricular tachyarrhythmias, and should be avoided if at all possible. Vasoconstrictors exacerbate peripheral vasoconstriction and reduce the effectiveness of passive warming techniques.

Tachyarrhythmias usually resolve with rewarming. Direct-current cardioversion may be ineffective while the patient remains hypothermic. Temporary pacing may be needed in cases of refractory bradycardia, but is usually not indicated.

Correction of acidosis is controversial as it may exacerbate alkalosis and further interfere with myocardial function.

Rewarming
Prevent further heat loss by moving into a warm environment as soon as possible and apply an insulating blanket. Such passive measures are sufficient in cases of mild hypothermia, with core temperature increasing by approximately 0.5°C per hour. Active measures may be indicated in more severe cases, and can be subdivided into methods that apply heat externally, and those that rewarm the core:

- Active external rewarming: methods include trunk immersion in a warm bath (40–45°C, or the warmest a conscious patient will tolerate), or the application of heated blankets (warm air blowers or electric blankets). More effective than passive measures, but peripheral vasodilation can induce both hypotension and a further drop in core temperature (the latter increasing the risk of arrhythmias).
- Active core rewarming: techniques include inhalation of warmed gases, peritoneal dialysis or hemodialysis, gastric or rectal lavage, and cardio-pulmonary bypass.

Such methods are invasive, but may be necessary, particularly in cases of refractory cardiac arrhythmias.

Treatment of cause/predisposing conditions
Unless the cause is obvious (eg, immersion, exposure), consider whether other conditions have contributed to the admission, including:
- drugs/alcohol
- other causes of coma
- major trauma
- hypothyroidism
- hypopituitarism.

Prognosis
Mortality rates vary from 20% to 85% according to age, chronic health state, degree of hypothermia, and rewarming/supportive treatment.

Heat stroke
Heat stroke is defined as hyperthermia associated with CNS dysfunction. It occurs when the body's capacity to lose heat is exceeded by heat production.

Pathophysiology
The principal physiologic response to a rise in core temperature is vasodilation. Heat is then delivered to the skin and lost by conduction and convection to the ambient air. The ability of such mechanisms to maintain a normal body temperature depends upon the ambient air temperature and its motion relative to the individual. Thus, convective and conductive losses cease at an air temperature over 32°C, and at even lower temperatures if the air is moving (eg, during exercise). Under such circumstances heat can be lost only by evaporation of sweat.

Temperature is a fundamental determinant of the rate of biochemical reactions, and as a result the physiologic consequences of a rise in body temperature are varied and widespread. Protein denaturation begins at 41°C, particularly vulnerable cells being elements of the cerebral and cerebellar cortex, vascular endothelium, renal and liver cells, and striated muscle.

Clinical features

Clinical features of heat stroke are shown in Figure 12.24. It presents with the classic triad of neurologic dysfunction, hyperthermia, and hot, dry skin.

Management

Investigations

Laboratory investigations to carry out the following:

- arterial blood gases
- complete blood count, clotting screen
- urea, electrolytes, blood sugar, liver function tests, calcium, and phosphate
- creatine kinase
- urinalysis (for myoglobinuria).

General support

Intubate and ventilate as indicated; the high minute ventilatory requirements must be maintained in order to avoid respiratory acidosis. Hypovolemia must be corrected as a reduction in peripheral perfusion due to hemodynamic collapse is followed by a rapid rise in core temperature. It is also important to correct metabolic disturbances. To support kidney function, mannitol may afford some renal protection in rhabdomyolysis. Dialysis may be required in severe cases.

Cooling

Hyperthermia is a medical emergency and prompt initiation of therapy to reduce core temperature is more important than the precise method. Shivering provoked by cooling may be treated with intravenous benzodiazepines. Tepid sponging, or water sprays with continuous fanning, promotes heat loss by evaporation. Maintenance of peripheral blood flow makes this a more effective treatment. Immersion in packed ice/cold water and/or cold wet blankets induces heat loss by conduction. A more rapid initial reduction in temperature is possible, although peripheral vasoconstriction may limit its effectiveness.

Clinical features of heat stroke

Cardiovascular	Central hypovolemia due to expansion of the peripheral vascular compartment Dehydration due to evaporative losses Increased cardiac output (3 L/min per °C) Myocardial injury and cardiovascular collapse (which results in evaporative failure and rapid rise in core temperature)
Hematologic	DIC, thrombocytopenia, leukocytosis
Metabolic	Respiratory alkalosis, progressing to metabolic acidosis. Consequences of tissue breakdown include: • hyperkalemia • hypocalcemia (binding to released proteins) • raised creatine kinase • hyperphosphatemia • hyperglycemia
Musculoskeletal	Muscle breakdown and rhabdomyolysis
Neurologic	Irritability, confusion, seizures, coma
Renal	Acute renal failure due to dehydration, cardiac failure, and rhabdomyolysis
Respiratory	Increased oxygen consumption, carbon dioxide production Hyperventilation Acute lung injury and ARDS

Figure 12.24 Clinical features of heat stroke. ARDS, acute respiratory distress syndrome; DIC, disseminated intravascular coagulation.

Prognosis

The mortality rate may be as high as 50%, particularly in elderly people or those who have suffered extensive liver or muscle injury. Approximately 10% of survivors have permanent neurologic damage.

Chapter 13

Toxicology

Imre Noth
University of Chicago, Chicago, IL, USA

Patients presenting with poison, both accidental and intentional, is common. Over 80% of individuals exposed to poisons require admission to the hospital, but fewer than 1% will require admission to the intensive care unit (ICU). Prompt diagnosis and treatment can reduce mortality and morbidity.

General principles

Supportive care is the basis of all treatment in poisoned patients. A medical history and physical examination can help direct which toxins or poisons are involved. It is important to seek out all sources of information because obtaining a history from an attempted suicide patient may be difficult. There may be deliberate misinformation in this setting. One must always assess for co-ingestions, as most patients who attempt suicide will use two or more toxins. Consider withdrawal from drugs as a possibility; alcohol or opiate withdrawal can often present to the ICU. Suspect nontoxicologic causes for altered mental status (ie, blunt trauma leading to a subdural hematoma can occur in patients suffering from alcohol intoxication). Discussion with a local poison control center can often provide useful insights given the large range of toxicologic emergencies.

Clinical assessment
Physical examination
Specific areas to focus on are: the neurologic, cardiovascular, respiratory, and skeletal systems, skin, and temperature.

Neurologic system

A thorough neurologic examination will help assess the severity of the poisoning and possibly suggest the type of poison. The following points should be considered:

- Depressed level of consciousness; coma is common but nonspecific.
- Pyramidal signs, ataxia, hypotonia, hyperreflexia, and extensor plantar responses may present in people exposed to tricyclic antidepressants (TCAs) or anticholinergic agents.
- Abnormal movements such as oculogyric crisis or choreoathetosis may indicate organophosphamides.
- Dilated pupils are seen in methanol and anticholinergic agents, and miosis is seen in organophosphamides and opiates.

Cardiovascular system

Many poisons will cause hemodynamic instability, possibly due to a metabolic acidosis, but there are some specific changes. Hypotension is seen in TCAs and β blockers, tachycardia with TCAs and anticholinergic agents, and bradycardia with β blockers, and digoxin.

Respiratory system

Hyperventilation may suggest metabolic acidosis. The decision to intubate and mechanically ventilate is determined by the level of consciousness, safety of the airway, and the respiratory assessment, which should include arterial blood gases. Aspiration of gastric contents is a real risk that often occurs before reaching the hospital.

Skeletal system

It is important to look for signs of trauma. Severe head injuries may be masked by overdoses. Compartment syndromes and rhabdomyolysis may develop in patients unconscious for some time.

Skin

A loss of consciousness may lead to development of pressure sores. Burns or blisters on the skin, especially the hands and face, suggest a corrosive agent.

Temperature

A prolonged coma can lead to hypothermia. Hyperthermia is a feature of poisoning with drugs such as anticholinergics, amphetamines, and methylene dioxymethylamphetamine (ecstasy).

Investigations

Specific poison assays are often unhelpful as absorption is variable and a poor guide to prognosis. As most management is based around symptomatic treatment, general investigations are more appropriate.

Nontoxicologic investigations

Urine

Myoglobin from rhabdomyolysis will color urine brown. Crystals may occur with primidone and ethylene glycol poisoning. Osmolality and pH may be used as a guide to treatment (eg, forced alkaline diuresis in salicylate poisoning).

Inspection of blood

Chocolate color suggests methemoglobinemia. Pink serum suggests hemolysis (eg, sodium chlorate poisoning). Rhabdomyolosis will release myglobin, resulting in brown serum.

Plasma osmolality

An osmolar gap discrepancy between measured and calculated plasma osmolality occurs with ethanol, methanol, and ethylene glycol poisoning.

Liver function

Alanine aminotransferase (ALT) >5,000 IU/L suggests acetaminophen/paracetamol or mushroom poisoning. A prolonged international normalized ratio (INR) suggests liver necrosis or warfarin overdose.

Serum potassium

Hypokalemia occurs with theophyllines and sympathomimetics. Hyperkalemia is often secondary to cell necrosis or cardiac glycosides.

Acid–base and arterial blood gas disturbances

Metabolic acidosis is very common, particularly with salicylates, acetaminophen/paracetamol, TCAs, carbon monoxide, cyanide, ethylene glycol, methanol, and iron. Respiratory alkalosis occurs with acid poisoning (eg, salicylates). Respiratory acidosis can occur as a result of depression of the central nervous system (CNS).

Hypoglycemia

Insulin or oral hypoglycemic agents will lower blood glucose. Hypoglycemia is secondary to severe liver necrosis.

Urea and creatinine

Renal function is often critical for the elimination of a poison. Acute renal failure may develop secondary to hypotension and hypovolemia, rhabdomyolysis, or liver failure. Heavy metals and ethylene glycol also cause acute renal failure.

EKG

Tachycardia with prolonged PR and QRS occurs in TCA poisoning. Depressed ST segments are seen in glycoside overdoses. and J waves in cases of hypothermia.

Chest and abdominal X-rays

Look for signs of pulmonary aspiration. Plain X-rays may reveal signs of heavy metal ingestion if taken in large quantities.

Toxicologic investigations

Assays for particular drugs are required urgently only if treatment is likely to change. Urine analysis is often better for use as a poison screen if the identity of the ingested substance is not known. Drugs that can be measured in the blood include carboxyhemoglobin, ethanol, ethylene glycol, methanol, barbiturates, iron, lithium, acetaminophen/paracetamol, theophylline, and salicylates.

Trial by antagonist

Flumazenil 0.5–1.0 mg i.v. and naloxone 0.2–0.4 mg i.v. will reverse benzo-diazepines and opioids, respectively, but have short half-lives and are therefore not often given by infusion for therapeutic purposes.

Management
Resuscitation

Resuscitation follows standard **A**irway, **B**reathing, **C**irculation protocols:

- **A**irway: unless the airway is protected by intubation, the patient should be nursed in the recovery position to avoid the risk of aspiration.
- **B**reathing: oxygen should be administered in high concentrations and the need for ventilation should be assessed clinically, aided by pulse oximetry and arterial blood gas measurement.
- **C**irculation: hypotension and arrhythmias require continuous EKG and invasive pressure monitoring. Inotropes and antiarrhythmics should be given as necessary.
- CNS: have high index of suspicion of head injury and treat seizures or convulsions as required.

- Hypothermia: should be treated as necessary. Treatments should focus on passive techniques if possible. Active re-warming with measures such as gastric and peritoneal lavage can cause vasodilation and hypotension. Hypothermia-induced cardiac arrest may be refractory until core temperature is restored. Malignant hyperthermia is life threatening; principles of treatment include mechanical ventilation, passive cooling and vasodilation, muscle relaxation, non-depolarizing neuromuscular blocking agents, and dantrolene 1–10 mg/kg i.v.
- Criteria for admission to the ICU: need for intubation/ventilation, seizures, no response to verbal stimuli, partial pressure of carbon dioxide >6 kPa (45 mmHg), cardiac rhythm other than sinus, second- or third-degree heart block, QRS duration >0.12 s, and cardiovascular instability requiring invasive monitoring and inotropes.

Active treatment

Measures to reduce absorption include the following:

- Gastric lavage: this has decreased in popularity unless performed within 1 hour of ingestion or when life-threatening quantities of poison have been ingested. Gastric lavage is contraindicated after ingestion of corrosive substances or petroleum (as it causes pneumonitis). Alcohol delays gastric emptying, so that lavage may be worthwhile later than otherwise anticipated. Prior intubation is essential if the protective airway reflexes are in doubt. Figure 13.1 recommends when delayed lavage should be undertaken.
- Forced emesis: there is little evidence of benefit. Ipecac is the only safe emetic, but dehydration can occur, particularly in children.
- Single-dose charcoal: 50 g orally or via nasogastric tube. Charcoal binds drugs in the bowel lumen and absorbs drugs from the blood. It may be of benefit some hours after ingestion. It also causes vomiting and constipation.

Measures to increase drug elimination
Forced alkaline diuresis

This has now become controversial, although traditionally it was considered suitable for salicylate, barbiturate, and phenoxyacetate herbicide poisoning. The procedure is carried out as follows:

1. Insert central venous pressure line and restore normal intravascular volume.
2. Give furosemide 20 mg i.v. if urine output <4 mL/min after fluid resuscitation.

Indications for delayed gastric lavage

Poison	Amount over	Within the previous
Aspirin	15 g	14 hours
Acetaminophen/paracetamol	10 g	4 hours
Benzodiazepines	Lavage not indicated unless massive overdose	Lavage not indicated unless massive overdose
Digoxin	5 g	8 hours
Tricyclics	750 mg	8 hours
Methanol	25 mL	8 hours
Ethylene glycol	100 mL	4 hours
Phenobarbital	1 g	8 hours
Phenytoin, valproate	Lavage not indicated unless massive overdose	Lavage not indicated unless massive overdose
Theophylline	25 g	4 hours (8 hours if slow release)
Dextropropoxphene	325 mg	8 hours

Figure 13.1 Indications for delayed gastric lavage.

3. Once urine output is established, rotate the following IV infusions:

1.26% sodium bicarbonate	500 mL
5% dextrose	500 mL
5% dextrose	500 mL
0.9% sodium chloride	500 mL

4. At initial rate of 1 L/h, reducing to 0.5 L/h after 6 h.
5. Replace K^+ losses as appropriate.
6. Monitor urine pH (aim for 7.5–8.5), hourly fluid balance, serum K^+. Check arterial blood gases 1- to 2-hourly, and salicylate levels 6-hourly.
7. Significant risk of pulmonary edema.

Forced acid diuresis

This increases phencyclidine and amphetamine elimination; however, it has no proven benefit.

Hemodialysis and hemoperfusion

These procedures (Figure 13.2) are useful in drugs with small volumes of distribution, and are necessary when renal function is poor. In many cases multiple dose-activated charcoal (MDAC) is as effective and less invasive. Hemodialysis and hemoperfusion should be reserved for life-threatening cases, particularly if renal function is impaired.

Poisonings where hemodialysis/perfusion may be of benefit	
Hemodialysis	**Hemoperfusion through charcoal**
Salicylates	Salicylates
Phenobarbital	Phenobarbital
Barbital	Barbital
Methanol and ethanol	Short- and medium-acting barbiturates
Ethylene glycol	Trichlorethanol derivatives
Lithium	Disopyramide
Isopropanol	Theophyllines
Carbamazepine	

Figure 13.2 Poisonings where hemodialysis/perfusion may be of benefit.

Multiple dose-activated charcoal

MDAC (Figure 13.3) reduces absorption and promotes elimination into the gastrointestinal tract. It is most efficacious with drugs with small volume distribution, low pK_a, low binding affinity, and long elimination half-life. In adults: 50 g orally followed by 50 g 4-hourly or 12.5 g hourly depending on vomiting. In children: 10–15 g initially then 4-hourly if tolerated. If the patient is compliant, continue until features of toxicity are resolved.

Role of multiple dose-activated charcoal in poisoning	
Drugs effectively bound by MDAC	**MDAC not effective for**
Alphachlorase	Acids/alkalis
Barbiturates	Cyanide
Carbamazepine	Ethanol
Chlormethiazole	Ethylene glycol
Dapsone	Iron
Digoxin	Lithium
Phenobarbital	Methanol
Phenytoin	
Quinine	
Salicylates	
Theophylline	

Figure 13.3 Role of multiple dose-activated charcoal in poisoning. MDAC, multiple dose-activated charcoal.

Role of multiple dose-activated charcoal in poisoning

Poison	Antidote
Acetaminophen/paracetamol	N-Acetylcysteine, methionine
Opioids	Naloxone
Benzodiazepines	Flumazenil
Carbon monoxide	(Hyperbaric) oxygen
Digoxin	Digoxin-specific Fab antibodies
β Blockers	Glucagon
Methanol, ethylene glycol	Ethanol
Organophosphates	Pralidoxime, atropine

Figure 13.4 Role of multiple dose-activated charcoal in poisoning.

Specific antidotes

There are a limited number of poisons that have specific antidotes (Figure 13.4). If the poison is known (Figure 13.5), careful and speedy use of the antidote will reduce morbidity. Many antidotes are toxic in their own right and should be reserved for life-threatening poisonings.

Specific details on the clinical features and management of poisoning

Poison	Clinical features	Management
Acetaminophen/paracetamol	Ingestion of 10 g or more can cause liver damage. Nausea and vomiting followed by features of liver failure. Liver damage results from excessive quantities of toxic paracetamol metabolites overwhelming the conjugating mechanisms that would normally protect the liver. Aminotransferase levels increase from 12 hours to peak at 3 days. Prothrombin time is a sensitive indicator of function. Plasma concentrations of 250 mg/L at 4 hours or 50 mg/L at 12 hours are usually associated with liver damage. Renal tubular necrosis occurs less commonly independent of hepatic injury	Charcoal is effective, as is lavage if performed within 4 hours of ingestion. NAC and methionine provide substrates for hepatic conjugation reactions, and therefore may limit the liver injury that would otherwise occur. They are most effective if given within 10 h of ingestion. Patients whose plasma acetaminophen/paracetamol concentrations are above the normal treatment line should be treated with intravenous NAC. High-risk patients (those on enzyme-inducing drugs such as alcohol, carbamazepine, phenytoin, rifampicin, barbiturates, or those who are malnourished) should be treated if their levels are above the high-risk treatment line Regimen for NAC treatment: 150 mg/kg in 200 mL 5% dextrose over 15 min i.v. then 50 mg/kg in 500 mL over 4 hours, then 100 mg/kg in 1,000 mL over 16 hours. If the patient presents >10 hours after ingestion commence full treatment but discontinue if paracetamol levels return low. If >24 hours, there is no contraindication to treatment but the benefit is unproven. In fulminant hepatic failure the last dose should be repeated until the patient recovers from encephalopathy Methionine: oral alternative, useful for pre-hospital care; 2.5 g at once followed by three further doses 4-hourly Liver transplantation: indications are a pH <7.3 or INR >6.5 plus creatinine >300 mmol/L or grade 3–4 encephalopathy

Figure 13.5 Specific details on the clinical features and management of poisoning. INR, international normalized ratio; NAC, N-acetylcysteine. (Continued on p.246–249).

Specific details on the clinical features and management of poisoning (continued)

Anticholinergics	Dilated pupils, no accommodation, dry mouth, ileus, urinary retention, agitation, delirium, hallucinations, convulsions, arrhythmias, hyperpyrexia	Supportive measures only needed. Physostigmine carries a significant risk of asystole
Aspirin	CNS: deafness, tinnitus, confusion, delirium, cerebral edema. Coma is rare but indicates severe poisoning. Cardiovascular: vasodilation, tachycardia, hypotension, cardiac arrest. Respiratory: hyperventilation, pulmonary edema. Vomiting, dehydration. Respiratory alkalosis followed by metabolic acidosis. Salicylate levels >700 mg/L indicate severe poisoning	Gastric lavage is effective up to 24 hours after ingestion as absorption is delayed. Activated charcoal and MDAC. Correct dehydration and acidosis. Forced alkaline diuresis is effective but high risk, particularly in elderly patients. Alkalinization of urine is recommended if plasma concentration >500 mg/L (3.6 mmol/L). Hemodialysis/charcoal hemoperfusion in severe cases (levels 700–1,000 mg/L)
Benzodiazepines	Often taken in combination with alcohol or other antidepressants. Drowsiness, ataxia, dysarthria, nystagmus, hypotension, respiratory depression, and coma	Mainly supportive therapy. Long half-lives and active metabolites mean that recovery is often prolonged. Flumazenil 0.5 mg over 1 min, repeated if no response, may be used for diagnostic purposes but is not currently recommended for therapeutic reversal due to its short half-life. Risk of arrhythmias and convulsions if flumazenil is given in the presence of tricyclics
Carbon monoxide	Affinity for Hb is 250 times that of O_2, also binding avidly to myoglobin, and cytochrome oxidases. Reduces oxygen carriage and causes tissue hypoxia. Features include headaches and coma, nausea and vomiting, hyperventilation, hypotension, increased muscle tone. Classically cherry pink skin, although cyanosis more common. HbCO levels >40% or coma indicates severe poisoning. Pulse oximeters over-read SaO_2 in such circumstances; a CO oximeter should be used to measure SaO_2 and HbCO levels	Therapy with high inspired oxygen concentrations speeds up clearance of HbCO. Several studies have demonstrated the benefit of hyperbaric oxygen therapy in patients with any symptoms of CO poisoning. Although the practicalities of transferring patients to a hyperbaric chamber mean that many units restrict themselves to normobaric ventilation with 100% O_2, even delayed hyberbaric therapy may be of benefit. Binding of CO to other heme proteins such as the cytochromes may persist after HbCO levels have fallen to normal

Figure 13.5 Specific details on the clinical features and management of poisoning (continued). CNS, central nervous system; CO, carbon monoxide; Hb, hemoglobin; MDAC, multiple dose-activated charcoal; O_2, oxygen; SaO_2, arterial oxygen saturation. (Continued on the next page).

Specific details on the clinical features and management of poisoning (*continued*)

Cyanide	A product of many industrial processes. Generated during combustion of synthetic fabrics (thereby complicating smoke-inhalation injuries). Inhibits cytochrome oxidase. Clinical features include anxiety, headache and weakness, cerebral edema, pulmonary edema, arrhythmias, metabolic acidosis, coma, cardiovascular collapse, and sudden death	Ventilate with 100% oxygen. Given specific antidote: 1. Sodium nitrite 10 mL 3% solution over 3 min followed by sodium thiosulphate 25 mL of 50% solution over 10 min, followed by 30–60 mg/kg per h. Sodium nitrite coverts Hb to metHb, which binds CN^-. Sodium thiosulphate converts cyanide to thiocyanate 2. Dicobalt edetate 300 mg (20 m/L) over 1 min, repeated ×2 if necessary. Follow immediately with 50 mL glucose 50%. Dicobalt edetate chelates CN^- to form non-toxic cobalt- and cobalto-cyanides 3. Hydroxycobalamin 100 mg/kg i.v.
Digoxin	Noncardiac features include nausea and vomiting, abdominal pain, visual disturbances, headache, fatigue, hallucinations, and coma. Heart block and tachyarrhythmias are possible. Refractory hyperkalemia may be seen. Severe toxicity if levels >10 µg/L	MDAC increases elimination. Correct any hypokalemia. Treat tachyarrhythmias with amiodarone or phenytoin. Transvenous pacing may be necessary to control symptomatic bradyarrhythmias. In severe and refractory cases digoxin-specific Fab antibody-binding fragments (6 mg/kg)
Ethylene glycol	Odorless inebriation, nausea and vomiting, convulsions and coma, tetany. Hyperosmolality and severe metabolic acidosis are due to oxalic acid. Oxalate crystalluria leads to acute renal failure	Oral of IV ethanol 0.6 g/kg loading dose followed by 100 mg/kg/hour to maintain blood concentration at 1 g/L (IV 5–10% solution, oral 20%). (Ethanol inhibits the metabolism of ethylene glycol to glycoaldehyde and glycolate.) Continue until all ethylene glycol is eliminated. Hemodialysis is indicated if levels >0.5 g/L or if more than 30 g has been ingested

Figure 13.5 Specific details on the clinical features and management of poisoning (*continued*). CN^-, cyanide; Hb, hemoglobin; MDAC, multiple dose-activated charcoal; metHb, methemoglobin. (*Continued overleaf*).

Specific details on the clinical features and management of poisoning (continued)

Heavy metals	Renal, hepatic, and GI damage is common	Supportive plus following specific antidotes: Mercury, arsenic: dimercaprol 2.5–5 mg/kg i.m. 4-hourly for 2 days, then 2.5 mg/kg i.m. twice a day for 2 weeks. Lead: sodium calcium edetate 50–70 mg/kg per day i.v. for 5 days Copper: penicillamine 0.25–2.0 g/day orally
Iron	Initial GI symptoms (nausea and vomiting, abdominal pain, GI bleeding) are followed by metabolic acidosis, coma, and shock. Liver necrosis may develop later. Pyloric and duodenal scarring may develop in the recovery phase, causing intestinal obstruction	MDAC not effective. Treatment with the iron-chelator desferrioxamine indicated if serum levels >5 mg/L or if poisoning dose >20 mg/kg. Protocol for treatment: 1. 2 g i.m. immediately 2. Leave 5 g in stomach lavage 3. IV infusion 5–15 mg/kg per h total to a maximum of 80 mg/kg per day (or 2 g i.m. twice a day)
Lead	GI symptoms, hepatorenal failure, convulsions, and coma	Treat as for heavy metals with dimercaprol and sodium calcium edetate
Lithium	Variety of GI and CNS disturbances, coma, hypotension and arrhythmias, hyponatremia and hypokalemia, nephrogenic diabetes insipidus. Mortality rate around 50%	Gastric lavage if within 1 hour of ingestion. Charcoal is ineffective. Slow absorption, therefore measure levels every 4–6 hours. Hemodialysis indicated in patients with CNS signs or levels >3.5–4 mmol/L
Methanol	Toxicity due to metabolism to formaldehyde and formic acid. Mild inebriation followed 8–36 hours later by GI symptoms, acidosis and coma. Decreasing visual acuity and dilated pupils precede blindness. Raised osmolality and increased anion gap	Use ethanol as for ethylene glycol (ethanol competitively inhibits metabolism of methanol). Correct acidosis. Hemodialyse if >30 g ingested or serum level >500 mg/L. Folinic acid 30 g may protect against blindness

Figure 13.5 Specific details on the clinical features and management of poisoning (continued). CNS, central nervous system; GI, gastrointestinal; MDAC, multiple dose-activated charcoal. (Continued on the next page).

Specific details on the clinical features and management of poisoning (*continued*)

Monoamine oxidase inhibitors	Features may take 12–24 hours to develop. Agitation, hyperreflexia convulsions, hyperpyrexia, and coma. Muscle spasms, trismus and rhabdomyolysis. Tachycardia and labile BP. Hypertensive crises unusual unless coincidental dietary abuse. Hyperthermia and hyperventilation	Supportive. Benzodiazepines to control agitation. Muscle paralysis and IPPV to relieve muscle spasms and help control hyperthermia. Fluids and vasopressors may be required to correct the relative hypovolemia and hypotension associated with vasodilation. β Blockers (phentolamine, phenoxybenzamine) and nitroprusside may help control hypertension
Paraquat	LD_{50} 3–5 g. Corrosive effects on upper respiratory and GI tracts. Pulmonary injury dominates early stages, is exacerbated by high oxygen tensions, and progresses to severe fibrosis. Multiple organ dysfunction is a common complication. Mortality rate up to 75%	General supportive therapy. After gastric lavage give 1 L 15% Fuller's earth suspension, followed by 20% mannitol. Keep FIO_2 as low as possible; extracorporeal oxygenation may help prevent pulmonary fibrosis. Hemodialysis is ineffective
Tricyclics	Symptoms appear within 4 hours, and include features of anticholinergic poisoning. EKG shows prolonged QT and QRS intervals	General supportive management. Single dose-activated charcoal 50–200 g. ICU if arrhythmias or prolonged EKG intervals. Correct acidosis. Sedate with benzodiazepines as necessary. Physostigmine treatment is short-lived, associated with arrhythmias, and is not recommended

Figure 13.5 Specific details on the clinical features and management of poisoning (*continued*). BP, blood pressure; EKG, electrocardiogram; FIO_2, fraction of inspired oxygen; ICU, intensive care unit; IPPV, intermittent positive pressure ventilation; LD_{50}, lethal dose 50% (ie, the dose of a chemical that kills 50% of the population).

Chapter 14

Scoring systems

John Kress
University of Chicago, Chicago, IL, USA

Severity of illness scoring systems are helpful for defining populations of critically ill patients because they facilitate, for example, comparison of different groups of patients enrolled in clinical trials. Such scoring systems may also guide more effective allocation of resources, such as nursing and ancillary care and help in assessing the quality of care in the intensive care unit (ICU) over time.

These scoring systems presume that increasing age, the presence of chronic medical illnesses, and increasingly severe derangements from normal

Points assigned to age and chronic disease as part of the APACHE II score	
Age (years)	**Score**
<45	0
45–54	2
55–64	3
65–74	5
≥75	6
History of chronic conditions	
None	0
Present	
Elective surgical patient	2
Emergency surgical or nonsurgical patient	5

Figure 14.1 Points assigned to age and chronic disease as part of the APACHE II score.
APACHE, Acute Physiology, Age, and Chronic Health Evaluation. The APACHE II score is the sum of the acute physiology, age, and chronic health points. Worst values during the first 24 h in the intensive care unit (ICU) should be used. Specific diagnostic categories have coefficients assigned to weight the score. APACHE II can be used for audit, research, and comparing outcomes. APACHE III, a commercially available computer program that calculates the APACHE II score, also takes into account the time of admission to the ICU and applies weighting to physiologic variables; it can provide an estimated risk of death for each patient.

Assignment of points in the Acute Physiology Score

	4	3	2	1	0	1	2	3	4
Rectal temperature (°C)	≥41.0	39.0–40.9	—	38.5–38.9	36.0–38.4	34.0–35.9	32.0–33.9	30.0–31.9	≤29.9
Mean blood pressure (mmHg)	≥160	130–159	110–129	—	70–109	—	50–69	—	≤49
Heart rate (ventricular response/min)	≥180	140–179	110–139	—	70–109	—	55–69	40–54	≤39
Respiratory rate (breaths/min) (spontaneous or mechanical)	≥50	35–49	—	25–34	12–24	10–11	6–9	—	≤5
Oxygenation (kPa):					—				
if FiO_2 >0.5 use $(A–a)DO_2$	—	≥500	350–499	200–349	<200	—	—	—	—
if FiO_2 <0.5 use PaO_2	—	—	—	—	>70	61–70	—	55–60	<55
Arterial pH	≥7.70	7.60–7.69	—	7.50–7.59	7.33–7.49	—	7.25–7.32	7.15–7.24	<7.15
Serum sodium (mmol/L)	≥180	160–179	155–159	150–154	130–149	—	120–129	111–119	≤110
Serum potassium (mmol/L)	≥7.0	6.0–6.9	—	5.5–5.9	3.5–5.4	3.0–3.4	2.5–2.9	—	<2.5
Serum creatinine (mg/100 mL)	≥3.5	2.0–3.4	1.5–1.9	—	0.6–1.4	—	<0.6	—	—
Hematocrit	≥60	—	50–59.9	46–49.9	30–45.9	—	20–29.9	—	<20
WBC count (×10^3/mL)	≥40	—	20–39.9	15–19.9	3–14.9	—	1–2.9	—	<1

Figure 14.2 Assignment of points in the Acute Physiology Score. $(A–a)DO_2$, difference in alveolar and arterial oxygen; FiO_2, inspired oxygen fraction; PaO_2, partial pressure of arterial oxygen; WBC, white blood cell count. To obtain the Glasgow Coma Scale (GCS) component, subtract the GCS from 15 to obtain the points assigned.

physiology are associated with increased mortality. All currently existing severity of illness scoring systems are derived from patients who have already been admitted to the ICU. There are no validated scoring systems to help triage ICU admission.

Acute Physiology and Chronic Health Evaluation (APACHE) II score

Currently, the most commonly utilized scoring system in North America is the APACHE (Acute Physiology and Chronic Health Evaluation) score (Figure 14.1). Age, type of ICU admission (eg, elective post-surgical vs non-surgical, or emergency post-surgical), a chronic health problem score, and the Acute Physiology Score (APS; Figure 14.2) are used to derive a score. The predicted hospital mortality is derived from a formula that takes into account the APACHE II score, the need for emergency surgery, and a weighted, disease-specific diagnostic category.

Organ system failure definitions

I. Cardiovascular failure (presence of one or more of the following):
    • Heart rate ≤54 beats/min
    • Mean arterial pressure ≤49 mmHg
    • Occurrence of ventricular tachycardia and/or ventricular fibrillation
    • Serum pH 7.24 with a $PaCO_2$ of 50 mmHg (6.7 kPa)

II. Respiratory failure (presence of one or more of the following):
    • Respiratory rate <5 breaths/min or >49 breaths/min
    • $PaCO_2$ ≥50 mmHg (6.7 kPa)
    • (A–a)DO_2 ≥350 mmHg
    • Dependency on mechanical ventilation ≥72 hours

III. Renal failure (presence of one or more of the following, excluding chronic dialysis before hospital admission):
    • Urine output <480 mL/24 h or <160 mL/8 h
    • Serum blood urea nitrogen ≥100 mg/100 mL
    • Serum creatinine ≥3.5 mg/100 mL

IV. Hematologic failure (presence of one or more of the following):
    • WBC ≤1 × 10⁹/L
    • Platelets ≤20 × 10⁹/L
    • Hematocrit ≤20%

V. Neurologic failure:
    • Severe head injury is defined as a GCS of 9 or less (in the absence of sedation at any one point in a day)
    • Coma is defined as 'no words, no eye opening, no response to commands' (ie, E1, V2, M5, or less)

Figure 14.3 Organ system failure definitions. (A–a)DO_2, difference in alveolar and arterial oxygen; FiO_2, inspired oxygen fraction; GCS, Glasgow Coma Scale; PaO_2, partial pressure of arterial oxygen; WBC, white blood cell count.

More recently, the APACHE III scoring system has been released, which is derived from a larger database than the APACHE II score, although the scoring system is otherwise similar. Unfortunately, severity of illness scoring systems lack the ability to predict survival in individual patients. Figure 14.3 shows the current definitions for organ system failure.

Chapter 15

Obstetric emergencies

Brian Gehlbach
University of Chicago, Chicago, IL, USA

Physiologic changes at term

Figures 15.1–15.4 highlight some of the physiologic changes that occur in pregnancy, namely:

- respiratory
- hematologic
- renal
- hemodynamics
- blood gas
- plasma protein changes.

Pre-eclampsia and eclampsia

Pre-eclampsia classically presents as the development of hypertension, proteinuria, and edema following week 20 of gestation. The risk is generally greatest near term and is increased by nulliparity, pre-existing hypertension or renal disease, diabetes mellitus, multiple gestation, hydatidiform mole, and antiphospholipid antibody syndrome. Progression to seizures (ie, eclampsia) or the HELLP syndrome (**h**emolysis, **e**levated **l**iver enzymes, and **l**ow **p**latelets) may occur suddenly, and is associated with a high rate of maternal and fetal complications, including death.

Definition of pre-eclampsia

The following characteristics define pre-eclampsia:

- gestation >20 weeks
- systolic blood pressure ≥140 mmHg or diastolic blood pressure ≥90 mmHg on two or more occasions, at least 4–6 hours (but not more than 7 days) apart, in a patient with previously normal blood pressure. An

Respiratory changes at term

Parameter	Change
Diaphragm excursion	Increased
Chest wall excursion	Decreased
Pulmonary resistance	Decreased 50%
Forced expiratory volume	None
Forced expiratory volume/forced vital capacity	None
Flow–volume loop	None
Closing capacity	None
Inspiratory reserve volume	+5%
Tidal volume	+45%
Expiratory reserve volume	−25%
Residual volume	−15%
Functional residual capacity	−20%
Vital capacity	None
Dead space	+45%
Respiratory rate	None
Minute ventilation	+45%

Figure 15.1 Respiratory changes at term.

Hematologic changes at term

Parameter	Change
Blood volume	+45%
Plasma volume	+55%
Red cell mass	+30%
Hemoglobin	−15%
Hematocrit	−15%
White cell count	Increased (polymorpholeukocytosis)
Prothrombin time	Shortened
Activated partial thromboplastin time	Shortened
Thromboelastography	Hypercoagulable
Platelet count	None/decreased
Bleeding time	Shortened
Fibrin degradation products	Increased
Fibrinogen	Increased
Plasminogen	Increased

Figure 15.2 Hematologic changes at term.

Renal changes and hemodynamics at term

Parameter	Change
Renal changes	
Glomerular filtration rate	Increased
Renal blood flow	Increased
Creatinine clearance	Increased
Plasma urea	Decreased
Plasma creatinine	Decreased
Hemodynamics	
Cardiac output	+50%
Stroke volume	+25%
Heart rate	+25%
Left ventricular end-diastolic volume	Increased
Ejection fraction	Increased
Pulmonary capillary wedge pressure	None
Central venous pressure	None
Systemic vascular resistance	−20%

Figure 15.3 Renal changes and hemodynamics at term.

Blood gas and plasma protein changes at term

Parameter	Nonpregnant	Term
Blood gas changes		
$PaCO_2$ (mmHg)	40 (5.3 kPa)	30 (4 kPa)
PaO_2 (mmHg)	100 (13.3 kPa)	103 (13.7 kPa)
pH	7.40	7.44
$[HCO_3^-]$ (mmol/L)	24	20
Plasma protein changes		
Total protein (g/dL)	7.8	7.0
Albumin (g/dL)	4.5	3.3
Globulin (g/dL)	3.3	3.7
Plasma cholinesterase	N/A	Reduced by 25%
Colloid osmotic pressure	27	22

Figure 15.4 Blood gas and plasma protein changes at term. HCO_3^-, hydrogen carbonate; $PaCO_2$, partial pressure of carbon dioxide; PaO_2, partial pressure of oxygen.

increase from baseline of 30 or 15 mmHg for systolic blood pressure or diastolic blood pressure, respectively, should prompt increased monitoring for pre-eclampsia, even at levels <140/90 mmHg. Proteinuria >300 mg in 24 hours or urine protein ≥1 g/L in two random specimens 4–6 hours apart

• edema.

Pre-eclampsia superimposed on chronic hypertension is characterized by an abrupt increase in blood pressure, new or worsening proteinuria, and thrombocytopenia and elevated liver enzymes.

Pathophysiology

The pathophysiology of pre-eclampsia has not been fully elucidated but is likely to be related to abnormal placentation and placental hypo-perfusion. The abnormal placenta may release factors that cause systemic endothelial dysfunction in the mother, including increased capillary permeability, vasospasm, and platelet consumption. Fetal growth impairment occurs with reduced placental perfusion.

Complications

There are several likely complications of pre-eclampsia and eclampsia, and they can be classified into the following categories:

• cardiovascular: hypertensive cardiac failure, reduced plasma volume ('contracted circulation')
• respiratory: pulmonary edema, acute respiratory distress syndrome (ARDS)
• renal: proteinuria ± hypoalbuminemia, renal failure
• central nervous system: hypertensive encephalopathy, cerebral ischemia or infarction, cerebral hemorrhage, cerebral edema, seizures
• blood: thrombocytopenia, disseminated intravascular coagulation (DIC), hemolysis
• liver: hemorrhage and necrosis, abnormal liver function tests
• fetus: intrauterine growth retardation, pre-term delivery, placental abruption.

Treatment

In severe pre-eclampsia or eclampsia the mainstay of treatment is delivery of the fetus.

Management of hypertensive crises

The following highlights the most appropriate drugs for managing hypertension in severe pre-eclampsia or eclampsia:

- hydralazine: initial bolus 5 mg i.v.; repeat at dose of 5–10 mg i.v. every 20–30 min. If the target blood pressure is not achieved after a total of 30 mg, another agent should be used
- labetalol: initial bolus 10 mg i.v.; administer additional bolus up to 40 mg every 10–20 min, and 1–2 mg/min infusion
- nicardipine or nimodipine: may be useful when unresponsive to hydralazine or labelalol.

Drugs that are absolutely contraindicated in pregnancy include angiotensin-converting enzyme inhibitors, while sodium nitroprusside and diuretics are both relatively contraindicated. The use of sodium nitroprusside, should be restricted for short periods of crises as it may cause fetal cyanide toxicity, and diuretics may have a detrimental effect on intravascular volume depletion.

Prevention and treatment of eclampsia

Magnesium sulfate is the agent of choice for eclampsia yet its role in preventing eclampsia remains controversial; however, the following can be used as a guide to dosage:

- loading dose: 4–6 g of 20% IV solution
- maintenance dose: 1–2 g/h infusion
- beware toxicity: it is important to check serum levels and adjust the dose accordingly for renal function, and to continue this for 24 hours after delivery. One should also aim for a serum level of 2–3 mmol/L. It is also important to monitor urine output, the patellar reflex, and respiratory status.

In the event of a cardiorespiratory arrest 1 g of 10% IV calcium gluconate can be administered.

Critical care pitfalls

The transition from mild pre-eclampsia to eclampsia may be rapid, and as many as a third of eclamptic seizures start in the post-partum period. There is also a risk of pulmonary or cerebral edema with injudicious fluid therapy. In general, however, fluids should be administered only in the case of oliguria. Nondepolarizing muscle relaxants are potentiated by magnesium sulfate.

HELLP syndrome

HELLP syndrome carries a high maternal and perinatal mortality. Women may present with nonspecific complaints, such as malaise, nausea, vomiting, right upper quadrant pain, and headache. In 20% of cases, hypertension is absent. Endothelial dysfunction with subsequent fibrin deposition leads to widespread organ hypoperfusion which can manifest as acute renal failure, ARDS, cerebral edema, liver necrosis/bleeding, uteroplacental insufficiency, and placental abruption. Laboratory studies may reveal a microangiopathic hemolytic anemia, elevated bilirubin and serum transaminases, thrombocytopenia, elevated lactate dehydrogenase (LDH), and DIC. Other than delivery of the fetus, treatment is supportive. Plasmapheresis has been advocated for those women with delayed recovery following delivery.

Tocolytic-induced pulmonary edema

β Agonists are commonly used to inhibit pre-term labor. Pulmonary edema complicating this therapy typically occurs during or shortly after discontinuation of tocolytics, and seems to occur more often in twin gestations. Sometimes fever is present, which may suggest the presence of infection. While the mechanisms underlying this disorder remain obscure, hypervolemia is probably a major contributor to the pathogenesis of this condition. Treatment includes discontinuation of tocolytics, oxygen, and diuresis.

Amniotic fluid embolism

Amniotic fluid embolism (AFE) generally occurs during or shortly after labor, although it has also been associated with first and second trimester abortions. Embolization of amniotic fluid to the maternal circulation may result in mechanical obstruction of the pulmonary arteries and stimulation of pulmonary endothelial factors, causing increased alveolar capillary leak and activation of the clotting cascades. AFE carries a high maternal mortality.

Clinical presentation

Patients with AFE may present with a sudden cardiovascular collapse, cyanosis, DIC, pulmonary edema or ARDS.

Diagnosis

Identification of AFE is usually from clinical presentation or made *post mortem*.

Treatment

It is important to utilize a lung protective strategy for mechanical ventilation and invasive hemodynamic monitoring, to guide fluid and vasoactive drug therapy. DIC may cause bleeding or thrombosis; the appropriate management of this condition is complex and may require a hematology consultation.

Acid aspiration syndrome

Pathogenesis

Aspiration of acidic gastric contents into the lungs stimulates bronchospasm and alveolar inflammation (pneumonitis), which may progress to ARDS. Predisposing factors in the obstetric patient include reduced integrity of the lower esophageal sphincter and a reduced rate of gastric emptying. Aspiration can occur during difficult/failed intubation, seizures, and other obstetric catastrophes.

Treatment of massive acid aspiration

Therapies for the acid aspiration include:

- endotracheal intubation
- tracheal suctioning
- mechanical ventilation using a lung-protective strategy and the least positive end-expiratory pressure (PEEP) that provides an adequate arterial oxygenation
- invasive monitoring may be required for hemodynamic instability.

The use of antibiotics is controversial, and some critical care units prefer to wait for evidence of infection before initiating antibiotic therapy. Corticosteroids have no proven benefit.

Prevention in high-risk patients

In patients who are at a considerably high risk for acid aspiration syndrome, there are a number of preventive measures that can be adopted:

- having a reasonable period of preoperative fasting
- utilizing preoperative H_2-receptor antagonists to reduce gastric acid pH and volume, and preoperative metoclopramide to increase lower esophageal sphincter tone
- applying cricoid pressure with a rapid sequence induction of general anesthesia prior to endotracheal intubation
- extubation in the patient, when awake, on her side and in the head-down position.

Status asthmaticus

The effects of pregnancy on asthma are variable, with one-third of patients showing improvement, one-third remaining stable, and one-third worsening. Current evidence suggests that fetal outcome is improved by optimal maternal asthma control, although the risk of pre-term labor may still be increased.

Treatment

When considering the management of asthma in pregnant women, the step approach generally applies. It is important to ensure adequate oxygenation, because even mild hypoxemia may be harmful to the fetus. Given the respiratory alkalosis of pregnancy, a partial pressure of carbon dioxide greater than 35 mmHg (4.7 kPa) may indicate impending ventilatory failure. Inhaled bronchodilators should be used when indicated; however, epinephrine causes uterine arterial vasoconstriction and should be avoided. While permissive hypercapnia strategies employed in the management of mechanically ventilated patients with status asthmaticus have been associated with reduced mortality, the effects of this strategy on the fetus have not been well studied. Acidosis should be avoided where possible.

Intubation and resuscitation in pregnancy

Critical care problems

Acidosis is stressful to the fetus, suggesting that appropriately prompt intubation and mechanical ventilation of pregnant women with respiratory failure are desirable. Intubation may be particularly difficult due to edema of the pharynx, larynx, and vocal folds. Aspiration of gastric contents is a risk, and early application of cricoid pressure should be considered before endotracheal intubation. Increased maternal oxygen consumption and decreased oxygen reserves increase the risk of hypoxemia during intubation. When the patient is supine, aortocaval compression by the gravid uterus impairs venous return; during resuscitation, either the patient should be tilted 30° laterally with a wedge under the right side or an assistant should manually displace the uterus to the left and cephalad. Vasopressors are needed in hemodynamic collapse due to epidural anesthesia. Emergency cesarean section should be performed if resuscitation is unsuccessful after 5 minutes.

Index

abdominal injuries 206–208
abdominal X-ray, poisoning 240
abscess, brain 177
acetaminophen poisoning 244(fig), 245(fig)
acetylcholine (ACh) receptor antibody assay 126
aciclovir 106(fig), 182
acid aspiration syndrome 261
acid-base balance 92–95
acid-base disturbances/disorders
  acute liver failure 166
  acute severe pancreatitis 168
  analysis 94
  biochemical features 93(fig)
  massive transfusion 190
  mechanical ventilation complication 62
  poisoning 239
acid pepsin 155
acromegaly 151
activated protein C 194
acute chest syndrome, sickle cell disease 187
acute hypoxemic respiratory failure (AHRF) 56, 67
acute lung injury (ALI) 67–69
  acute respiratory distress syndrome vs. 68(fig)
  clinical features 68
  definition 67
  etiology 68(fig)
  management 68–69
acute myocardial infarction (AMI) 41–50
  biochemical changes 44
  EKG changes 42–44, 43(fig)
  management 45–50
    complications 47–50
    immediate 45–47
  medical examination 42
  medical history 42

  pathogenesis 41–42
  signs 42
  ST changes 42–43, 43(fig)
  temporary pacing indications 49
acute-on-chronic respiratory failure 85
Acute Physiology and Chronic Health Evaluation II (APACHE II) score 251(fig), 253–254
Acute Physiology Score (APS) 252(fig)
acute renal failure (ARF) 97–107
  acidosis treatment 101
  acute renal support 102–107
  classification 97–98
  definition 97
  diagnosis 98–99
  drug treatment 104, 106–107(fig)
  intrinsic 98
    causes 98
    prerenal vs. 99(fig)
    treatment 100–102
  laboratory abnormalities 99
  poisoning 240
  postrenal 98
  prerenal 97–98
    causes 97–98
    intrinsic vs. 99(fig)
    treatment 99–100, 100(fig)
  treatment 99–102
acute respiratory distress syndrome (ARDS) 67–69
  acute lung injury vs. 68(fig)
  clinical features 68
  definition 67
  etiology 68(fig)
  management 68–69
  neuromuscular blockade 10
  sickle cell disease 187
addisonian crisis 150

Addison's disease 149
adenosine 32(fig)
adrenergic blocking drugs 27, 28(fig)
adrenocortical insufficiency 149–151
    causes 149
    clinical features 149–150
    diagnosis 150
    management 150
adrenocorticotropic hormone (ACTH) 149
    secondary deficiency 149
adrenocorticotropic hormone (ACTH)
        stimulation test 150
adrenoreceptors 25(fig)
Advanced Cardiac Life Support (ACLS)
        guidelines 35, 36(fig)
advance directives 6
airway edema, smoke inhalation 225
airway management
    hypothermia 233
    near drowning 230
    poisoning 240
    spinal cord injury 209–211, 212(fig)
    status epilepticus 132
    tetanus 128
    trauma 203, 204(fig)
akinetic (atonic) seizure 132(fig)
albuterol 101
aldosterone 149
α_1-adrenoreceptors 25(fig)
alteplase (rt-PA)
    acute myocardial infarction 46
    acute renal failure 107(fig)
alveolar edema 56, 67
alveolar hemorrhage 67
amikacin 180
amino acids, parenteral nutrition 200
aminoglycosides 106(fig), 180
aminosteroid relaxants, tetanus 11
amiodarone 32(fig)
    acute renal failure 106(fig)
    atrial fibrillation 29
amniotic fluid embolism (AFE) 260–261
    clinical presentation 260
    diagnosis 260
    treatment 261
amphotericin 182
    acute renal failure 106(fig)
    pneumonia, immunocompromised host 78
ampicillin 178
    bacterial meningitis 138(fig), 139(fig)
analgesia 7–13
    burns 224

drug types 7–11
    indications 7
    see also individual drugs
anesthetic agents
    brain herniation 113
    intravenous see intravenous anesthetic
        agents
aneurysm 50
angina, unstable 40–41
    definition 40
    high risk predictors 41
    management 41
    surgical management 41
angiography
    acute myocardial infarction 45
    pulmonary embolism 89
    unstable angina 41
angiotensin-converting enzyme inhibitors
        (ACEIs) 30 (fig)
    acute renal failure 106(fig)
    heart failure 40
anion gap 94–95
    metabolic acidosis 94–95
    normal 94
antacid therapy 168
antecubital fossa catheterization 16(fig)
anterior cord syndrome 209(fig)
anterior spinal artery syndrome 209(fig)
anthrax 178
antiarrhythmic drugs 32–34(fig)
    acute renal failure 106(fig)
    thyrotoxic crisis 148
    Vaughan-Williams classification 31(fig)
antibiotics 178–181
    acute renal failure 106(fig)
    acute severe pancreatitis 169
    bacterial meningitis 138(fig), 139(fig)
    chronic obstructive pulmonary disease 86
    community-acquired pneumonia 72–73,
        74–75(fig)
        treatment failure 72–73
    endocarditis 177
    gastric acid aspiration 80
    hospital-acquired pneumonia 77(fig), 174,
        175(fig)
    ventilator-associated pneumonia 174,
        175(fig)
    see also individual drugs
anticholinergics, poisoning 246 (fig)
anticholinesterase therapy 127
anticoagulation
    acute myocardial infarction 47

hemodialysis 103
pulmonary embolism 90
antidiuretic hormone (ADH)
diabetes insipidus 134
syndrome of inappropriate antidiuretic
hormone secretion 136
antidotes 244, 244(fig), 245–249(fig)
antifibrinolytics 195
antifungals 106(fig), 182–183
antithyroid treatment 148
antituberculous drugs 106(fig)
antivirals 106(fig), 182
aorta, ruptured 207(fig)
APACHE II score 251(fig), 253–254
APACHE III score 254
aprotinin 195
argatroban 90
Argyll Robertson pupils 110
arrhythmias 29, 31–35
acute myocardial infarction 48
causes 29
see also individual types
arterial oxygen content 55
arterial pressure monitoring 15–16
artificial ventilation, traumatic brain injury
118
aspartate transaminase (AST) 44
aspiration syndromes 79–81
etiology 79
pathophysiology 80–81
aspirin
acute myocardial infarction 46
poisoning 246 (fig)
unstable angina 41
assist-control ventilation 63
asthma, acute severe 82–84
features 82
see also status asthmaticus
atenolol 28(fig), 47
atonic (akinetic) seizure 132(fig)
atracurium 11
cis-atracurium 11
atrial fibrillation 29
atrial flutter 31
acute myocardial infarction 48
atrial tachycardia 31
autonomic hyperreflexia 215
AVPU scheme 208
awake fiberoptic intubation
smoke inhalation 226
spinal cord injury 211
azathioprine 107(fig), 127

azithromycin 74(fig), 75(fig)
aztreonam 180

Bacillus anthracis 178
bacterial translocation, peptic erosion 155
balloon tamponade 161–162
barbiturate coma 118
basilic vein catheterization 16(fig)
bat-wing edema 39
benzodiazepines 9, 9(fig)
acute renal failure 106(fig)
poisoning 246(fig)
tetanus 129
benzylpenicillin 178
pneumonia 75(fig)
β_1-adrenoreceptors 25(fig)
β_2-adrenoreceptors 25(fig)
β_2 agonists 82, 83
β blockers
acute myocardial infarction 46–47
acute renal failure 106(fig)
thyrotoxic crisis 148
unstable angina 41
β-lactamase 77(fig)
β-lactams 180
hospital-acquired pneumonia 77(fig)
bicarbonate 93
bisphosphonates 154
biventricular failure 37
blood, endogenous vs. stored 189
blood count, community-acquired pneumonia
71
blood culture, community-acquired
pneumonia 71
blood gas analysers 94
blood gas analysis 92–95
carbon monoxide poisoning 227
community-acquired pneumonia 71
poisoning 239
term pregnancy 259(fig)
blood inspection, poisoning 239
blood loss, hemodynamic features 206(fig)
blue asphyxia 219(fig)
botulism 129–130
clinical features 129–130
diagnosis 130
differential diagnosis 130
management 130
prognosis 130
types 129
bradyarrhythmias, organ donors 123
bradycardias 48–49

brain abscess 177
brain death 119–121
  diagnostic criteria 119–121
    absent brain-stem function 120,
      121(fig)
    absent cerebral function 119
    irreversibility 120–121
    diagnostic tests 121(fig)
brain herniation 113–115
  management 113, 115
  syndromes 114(fig)
brain injury
  secondary 115(fig)
  traumatic see traumatic brain injury (TBI)
brain-stem reflex testing 120, 121(fig)
bretyllium 32(fig)
bronchitis, chronic 86(fig)
bronchodilators 82, 86, 191, 262
Brown–Séquard syndrome 209(fig)
buccal nitrate 41
buffer 92
buffering systems, biologic 92–94
bundle-branch block, acute myocardial
    infarction 48–49
burns 219–225
  analgesia 224
  depth 220, 222(fig)
  fluid resuscitation 220, 222–223
  management 220, 222–225
    circulation 220, 222–223
    respiratory care 220
  nutritional support 224–225
  pathophysiology 219–220, 221(fig)
  prognosis 225
  size assessment 220
  wound management 224
burns shock 219, 232

cachexia 197
calcitonin 154
calcitriol 153
calcium channel blockers 30(fig)
calcium chloride 153
calcium gluconate 101, 152
calcium-losing states 151–152
calcium supplementation, hypocalcemia 152
calciuresis 154
capnography 58–59, 58(fig)
captopril 30(fig)
carbon monoxide poisoning 227–228
  clinical features 227, 246(fig)
  treatment 227, 244(fig), 246(fig)

cardiac arrest, resuscitation guidelines 35,
    36(fig)
cardiac enzymes
  acute myocardial infarction 44
  heart failure 39
cardiac failure see heart failure
cardiac injuries, penetrating 207(fig)
cardiac massage, hypothermia 233
cardiac tamponade 207(fig)
  acute myocardial infarction 49
cardiogenic shock 50–52
  acute myocardial infarction 49
  causes 50
  clinical features 50–51
  definition 50
  hemodynamic profile 27(fig)
  management 51–52
  outcome 52
  surgical revascularization 52
cardiomegaly 38
cardiopulmonary resuscitation (CPR), near
    drowning 231
cardiothoracic injuries, traumatic 207(fig)
cardiovascular failure, definition 253(fig)
cardiovascular system 15–52
  acute severe pancreatitis 168
  burns 221(fig)
  hypothermia 232(fig)
  inotropic support 24–25
  mechanical ventilation indications 62
  near drowning 229(fig)
  noninvasive monitoring 22–23
  poisoning 238
  pressure monitoring 15–16
    damping 15
    resonance 15
    transducer systems 15
    tubing kinks/clots 15
    zero errors 15
  spinal cord injury 213–214
  see also individual diseases/disorders
care provision, exemplary 1–6
caspofungin 183
catecholamines 24, 25(fig), 26(fig)
  cardiogenic shock 51
catheter/catheterization
  antecubital fossa 16(fig)
  basilic vein 16(fig)
  central venous see central venous
catheterization
  external jugular vein 16(fig)
  femoral vein 16(fig)

pulmonary artery *see* pulmonary artery
   catheters (PACs)
pulmonary artery flotation catheter 20, 168
subclavian vein 16(fig)
cefazolin 77(fig), 179
cefotaxime 179
   bacterial meningitis 138(fig), 139(fig)
   pneumonia 74(fig)
ceftazidime 179
ceftriaxone 74(fig), 75(fig), 139(fig)
cefuroxime 77, 179
central cord syndrome 209(fig)
central nervous system (CNS)
   dysfunction assessment 208
   mechanical ventilation indications 62
   poisoning 240
   traumatic injury 206
central venous catheterization 16–18
   cardiogenic shock 51
   central venous pressure measurement
      17–18, 18(fig)
   complications 17(fig)
   hypothermia 233
   indications 17
   insertion sites 16(fig)
   parenteral nutrition administration 200–201
central venous pressure (CVP)
   interpretation 17, 18
   measurement 17–18, 18(fig)
   right ventricular end-diastolic volume
   relationship 17, 19(fig)
cephalosporin(s) 179
   acute renal failure 106(fig)
   hospital-acquired pneumonia 77(fig)
   pneumonia, immunocompromised host 78
cerebral edema 165
cerebral perfusion pressure 112
   maintenance 113, 117–118
cerebral salt wasting 136
   clinical features 135(fig)
   treatment 135(fig)
cerebrospinal fluid (CSF)
   abnormalities 138(fig)
   buffering capacity, mechanical ventilation 62
   normal properties 137(fig)
   variations 137(fig)
cesarean section, emergency 262
chemical pneumonitis 80
chest physiotherapy, pneumonia 72
chest X-ray 53–55
   acute heart failure 38
   community-acquired pneumonia 70

lung parenchyma evaluation 55
lung volume changes 55
Pneumocystis jiroveci pneumonia 78–79
pneumonia 78(fig)
poisoning 240
pulmonary embolism 89
pulmonary tuberculosis 76
respiratory system evaluation 53–55
children, Glasgow Coma Scale 109, 111(fig)
Chlamydia psittaci 74(fig)
chronic obstructive pulmonary disease
   (COPD), acute deteriorations 85–87
   cardiorespiratory arrest 86–87
   clinical features 86(fig)
   management 85–87
   pathophysiology 85
   positive airway pressure 86
   respiratory failure 85
ciclosporin 107(fig)
cimetidine 157(fig)
ciprofloxacin 180–181
   acute renal failure 106(fig)
   pneumonia 74(fig)
circulation
   burns 220, 222–223
   clinical assessment 205
   hypothermia 233
   monitoring 205
   near drowning 230
   spinal cord injury (SCI) 213–214
circulatory support, nonpharmacologic
   24–25
clarithromycin 106(fig)
clindamycin 79
clinical hypotheses
   formulating 2
   testing 2
clinical skills
   development 2
   trusting 2
Clostridium botulinum 129
Clostridium tenani 128
clotting factors
   disseminated intravascular coagulation 194
   massive transfusion 189
coagulopathy, acute liver failure 166–167
co-amoxiclav 77(fig)
codeine 107(fig)
cold caloric vestibuloocular reflex 122(fig)
community-acquired pneumonia 69–73
   antibiotics 72–73, 74–75(fig)
   atypical 70

classification 70
clinical features 69–70
forms 74–75(fig)
ICU transfer indications 71–72
investigations 70–71
management 72
microbiology 71
monitoring 72
mortality 69
severe 70, 72
severity assessment 70
complete AV block 48
complex partial seizure 132(fig)
computed tomography (CT)
brain herniation 115
panhypopituitarism 151
pulmonary embolism 89
traumatic brain injury 115
consent 6
consolidation
physical signs 53(fig)
radiological appearance 54(fig)
continuous positive airway pressure (CPAP) 64
controlled mandatory ventilation (CMV) 63
cooling, heat stroke 235
cord hemisection 209(fig)
coronary angiography, acute myocardial
infarction 45
cor pulmonale, sickle cell disease 187
corticosteroids 148
cortisol 149
cough reflex, impaired 79
Coxiella burnetii 74(fig)
creatine kinase (CK) 44
creatinine 240
cricothyroidotomy, emergency 211
critical care, approaches to 1–6
critical care team 3
cryoprecipitate 194
crystalloid
burns 224(fig)
traumatic brain injury 117
Cullen's sign 167
cultures
community-acquired pneumonia 71
diabetic ketoacidosis 144
current (electrical) 216–217
cyanide poisoning 228, 247(fig)

d-dimers, pulmonary embolism 88
dead space fraction 56
Deamino-D-arginine vasopressin (DDAVP) 123

deep burns 222(fig)
deep vein thrombosis (DVT)
identification 89
pulmonary embolism 87
traumatic brain injury 119
dehydration, hyperosmolar nonketotic coma
144
desmopressin 123
devices, use discontinuation 2–3
dexamethasone
bacterial meningitis 139
cerebral edema 113
dexmedetomidine 10(fig)
dextropropoxyphene 107(fig)
dextrose
diabetic ketoacidosis 143
myxedema coma 147
diabetes insipidus (DI) 134
causes 136(fig)
clinical features 135(fig)
nephrogenic 134
neurogenic 134
organ donors 123
treatment 135(fig)
diabetic ketoacidosis (DKA) 141–144
causes 141, 142(fig)
clinical features 141–142
complications 144
laboratory findings 142
management 142–144
pathophysiology 142(fig)
diagnostic peritoneal lavage (DPL) 206
diarrhea, enteral nutrition complication 199
diazepam
properties 9(fig)
status epilepticus 133(fig)
digoxin 33(fig)
acute renal failure 106(fig)
atrial fibrillation 29
poisoning 244(fig), 247(fig)
thyrotoxic crisis 148
dihydrocodeine 107(fig)
2,3-diphosphoglycerate (2,3-DPG) 190
disopyramide 33(fig)
disseminated intravascular coagulation (DIC)
192–195
bleeding 193
causes 193
clinical features 193
differential diagnosis 193
laboratory diagnosis 193
management 193–194

organ dysfunction 193
thrombosis 193
traumatic brain injury 119
diuretics
acute renal failure 106(fig)
cerebral edema 113
chronic obstructive pulmonary disease 86
heart failure 40
diving reflex 228
dobutamine 26(fig), 40
'do no harm' 3
dopamine 26(fig)
dopexamine 26(fig)
Doppler flow measurement 22
doxycycline 74(fig)
Dressler syndrome 50
drowning
dry 228
near see near drowning
dysequilibrium syndrome 103

echocardiography 23
acute myocardial infarction 45
cardiogenic shock 51
heart failure 39
pulmonary embolism 89
transesophageal 23
transthoracic 23
eclampsia 255
complications 258
critical care pitfalls 259
prevention 259
treatment 258–259
edrophonium test 126
electrical injury 216–219
consequences 217
types 217–219
electrocardiography (EKG)
acute myocardial infarction 42–44, 43(fig)
heart failure 38–39
hyperkalemia 101
myxedema coma 146
poisoning 240
pulmonary embolism 89
'saddle-shaped' ST elevation 49
'saw-tooth' waves 31
electroencephalogram (EEG) 112
electrolyte resuscitation, diabetic
ketoacidosis 143
electrolytes
community-acquired pneumonia 71
massive transfusion 190

electromyogram (EMG), myasthenia gravis 126
embolism
amniotic fluid see amniotic fluid embolism
(AFE)
fat see fat embolism
pulmonary see pulmonary embolism (PE)
systemic 49, 207(fig)
emesis, forced 241
emphysema 86(fig)
enalapril 30(fig)
encephalopathy
acute liver failure complication 165
bleeding esophageal varices 161
classification 165(fig)
management 161
portosystemic shunting 162
endocarditis 177
endocrine system 141–154
see also specific disorders
endoscopic sclerotherapy 161
endoscopy, pancreatitis 169
endotracheal intubation
chronic obstructive pulmonary disease 86–87
complications 63
smoke inhalation 226
energy requirements 197
parenteral nutrition 197, 200
enteral nutrition 198–200
absorption failure 199
administration 199
advantages 198–199
complications 199–200
stress ulceration prevention 158
traumatic brain injury 118–119
Enterobacteriaceae 176(fig)
enterochromaffin-like (ECL) cells 156
Enterococcus faecalis 176(fig), 177
epilepsy 130–134
see also status epilepticus
epinephrine
clinical effects 26(fig)
status asthmaticus 84
equine serum botulism antitoxin 130
erythromycin 106(fig), 181
Escherichia coli 73, 74(fig), 77(fig), 138(fig)
esmolol 28(fig), 148
esomeprazole 157(fig)
esophageal Doppler monitoring (EDM) 22–23
esophageal transection 162
esophageal varices, bleeding 160–162
definition 160
management 160–162

ethambutol 78, 106(fig)
ethylene glycol poisoning 244(fig), 247(fig)
exemplary care provision 1–6
exposure 208
external jugular vein catheterization 16(fig)
extremities, hypothermia 232(fig)
extubation 66

facemasks 60, 61(fig)
family
  death management 4–5
  as surrogate decision-makers 6
famotidine 157(fig)
fat, parenteral nutrition 200
fat embolism 81–82
  causes 81
  clinical features 82
  cutaneous manifestations 81
  diagnosis 82
  management 82
  prognosis 82
femoral vein catheterization 16(fig)
fenoldopam 30 (fig)
fentanyl 8 (fig)
fiberoptic bronchoscopy, smoke inhalation 226
fibrin clot formation 192, 192(fig)
first degree burns 222(fig)
flecainide 33(fig)
fluconazole 106(fig), 183
flucytosine 183
fluid balance, intrinsic renal failure 100
fluid challenges 19(fig)
fluid replacement, pancreatitis 168
fluid restriction/diuresis, ARDS 69
fluid resuscitation
  burns 220, 222–223
    problems 222
  diabetic ketoacidosis 143
flumazenil 240
forced acid diuresis 242
forced alkaline diuresis 241–242
forced emesis 241
foscarnet 182
fosphenytoin 133(fig)
fractional excretion of Na⁺ (FE_{Na+}), acute renal failure 99
fractional excretion of urea, acute renal failure 99
fractures, blood loss 206(fig)
fresh frozen plasma, warfarin reversal 91
frostbite 232(fig)

full thickness burns 222(fig)
fungal infection 176(fig)
furosemide 106(fig), 113

gag reflex
  absence, brain death 121(fig)
  aspiration syndromes 79
ganciclovir 182
gas exchange defects
  causes 205(fig)
  pulmonary embolism 88
gas trapping, status asthmaticus 83–84, 84(fig)
gastric acid
  production 156
  suppression 156–158, 157(fig)
gastric acid aspiration 80
gastric ileus 199
gastric lavage 241, 242(fig)
gastric tonometry 159, 160(fig)
gastrin 156
gastro-esophageal aspiration 200
gastro-esophageal reflux, enteral nutrition 200
gastrointestinal disorders 155–170
  see also specific disorders
gastrointestinal integrity 155–160
  bleeding, high risk patients 159
  ICU management 156–158
  stress-related mucosal damage 155
    causes 156
    mechanisms 155
gastrostomy, percutaneous 199
G cells 156
generalized absence seizure 132(fig)
genitourinary system, spinal cord injury 216(fig)
gentamicin 180
  bacterial meningitis 139(fig)
gigantism 151
Glasgow Coma Scale (GCS) 109, 110(fig)
  modification for children 109, 111(fig)
glucose 101
glutamine supplementation 197–198, 200
glyceryl trinitrate (GTN) 30(fig)
  unstable angina 41
Gram-negative bacteria
  hospital-acquired pneumonia 73, 173
  nosocomial bacteremia 176(fig)
  pneumonia 74(fig)
Gram-positive bacteria, hospital-acquired pneumonia 73
Graves' disease 147

Grey Turner's sign 167
Guillain-Barré syndrome 124–125
  clinical features 124
  complications 125
  diagnosis 124
  differential diagnosis 124
  management 124–125
  predisposing factors 124
  prognosis 125

H_2-receptor blockers 156–157, 157(fig)
  acute liver failure 166
haloperidol 10(fig)
headache, raised intracranial pressure 113
health-care-associated pneumonia (HCAP) 73
heart and lung donors 122(fig)
heart block, acute myocardial infarction 48–49
heart donors 122(fig)
heart failure
  acute 35, 37–40
    clinical features 37–38
    investigations 38–39
    management 39–40
    pulmonary embolism 88
    signs 38
    symptoms 38
  acute myocardial infarction 49
  assessment 39
  causes 37
  chronic 35
  classification 35, 37
  hemodynamic profile 27(fig)
  inotropic support 40
heated blankets, hypothermia 234
heat loss, burns 221(fig)
heat stroke 234–236
  clinical features 235, 236(fig)
  definition 234
  laboratory investigations 235
  management 235
  pathophysiology 234–235
  prognosis 236
heavy metals, poisoning 248(fig)
Heimlich maneuver 80
heliox 84
HELLP syndrome 260
hematologic emergencies 185–195
  see also individual diseases
hematologic failure, definition 253(fig)
hematology
  heart failure 39
  term pregnancy 258–259(fig)

hemodialysis
  continuous 103, 105(fig)
  indications 102
  intermittent 103, 104(fig)
  poisoning 242
  problems/complications 103
hemodynamics
  blood loss 206(fig)
  cardiogenic shock 51–52
  mechanical ventilation 62
  pulmonary artery catheters 21
  shock states 27(fig)
hemoglobin, adult (HbA) 185
hemoglobin electrophoresis 186
hemoglobin S (HbS) 185
hemolytic anemia 186
hemoperfusion, poisoning 242
Hemophilus 70, 77(fig), 187
Hemophilus influenzae 74(fig), 188
hemostatic failure, massive transfusion 189
hemothorax 207(fig)
Henderson–Hasselbalch equation 93, 159
heparin
  acute myocardial infarction 47
  disseminated intravascular coagulation 194
  pulmonary embolism 90
  unstable angina 41
hepatitis, viral 163
herpes simplex virus 163, 182
herpes zoster virus 163, 182
high-output heart failure 37
high-tension injuries 217, 218
history taking 2
HIV, pneumonia 78
Holmes–Adie syndrome 110
hospital-acquired pneumonia (HAP) 73, 75,
    172–175
  antibiotics 77(fig), 174, 175(fig)
  clinical features 173
  definition 73
  diagnosis 73, 75, 76(fig), 173–174
  management 75, 77(fig), 174, 175(fig)
  multidrug-resistant pathogen risk factors
    174
  organisms 73
  risk factors 173
  traumatic brain injury 118
human albumin solution (HAS) 224, 224(fig)
human-derived botulinum antitoxin 130
human tetanus immunoglobulin (hTIG) 129
hydralazine 30(fig), 259
hydrocarbon aspiration 81

hyperacute fulminant asthma 82
hyperbaric oxygen therapy 227–228
hypercalcemia 153–154
  causes 153
  clinical features 153
  investigations 153–154
  management 154
hypercatabolic response 197
  burns 221(fig)
  starvation vs. 198(fig)
hyperdynamic shock 166
hyperglycemia 144
hyperkalemia
  massive transfusion 190
  treatment 101
hypermetabolic state, burns 221(fig)
hyperosmolar nonketotic coma
      144–145
  clinical features 144
  management 145
hypertension 27–29
hypertensive crises
  eclampsia 259
  pre-eclampsia 259
hyperthermia, poisoning 238
hypocalcemia 151–153
  causes 151–152
  clinical features 152
  investigations 152
  treatment 152–153
hypofibrinogenemia 194
hypoglycemia
  acute liver failure 166
  myxedema coma 147
  poisoning 239
hypokalemia
  acute liver failure 166
  massive transfusion 190
hyponatremia
  management 136
  myxedema coma 147
hypophosphatemia 154
hypotension
  organ donors 122
  trauma 205
hypotensive agents 27–29, 28 (fig)
hypothalamic disorders 136
hypothermia 231–234
  accidental 231
  classification 231(fig)
  definition 231
  diagnosis 231, 233

  management 233–234
    airway 233
    breathing 233
    circulation 233
    rewarming 233–234
  massive transfusion 189
  myxedema coma 147
  pathophysiology 232(fig)
  poisoning 238, 241
  prognosis 234
  tachyarrhythmias 233
  treatment of cause 234
hypovolemia
  hemodynamic profile 27(fig)
  organ donors 123
  prerenal acute renal failure 97
hypovolemic shock
  abdominal injuries 206
  burns 221(fig)
  fluid management 207
hypoxemia
  hemodialysis induced 103
  mechanisms 56
hypoxia 55

imipenem 106(fig), 180
immersion 228, 230(fig)
immobilization, spinal cord injury 209, 215,
      215(fig)
immunosuppressants 107(fig)
infection 171–183
  predisposing factors 173(fig)
  sickle cell disease 187, 188
  sites 172
  see also individual infections
inferior vena caval filters 92
inflammation 171–183
  acute 171(fig)
influenza virus 75(fig)
inhalational anthrax 178
inoconstrictors 24
inodilators 24, 52
inotropes 24, 233
inotropic support 24–25
  heart failure 40
insulating blankets, hypothermia 233
insulin 141
  deficiency, diabetic ketoacidosis 141, 142(fig)
  hyperkalemia 101
insulin therapy
  diabetic ketoacidosis 143–144
  intensive 145

intensive care unit (ICU)
  cost savings 4
  death management 4–5
    cure-comfort process switch 5, 5 (fig)
    experience of 5
    family 4–5
    patient 4
  economics 3–4
  human resources 4
  life-sustaining measures, withdrawal 5
  quality 5–6, 6 (fig)
  survival rates 4
internal jugular vein catheterization 16(fig)
interstitial edema 38
intervention minimization 3
intestinal fluid aspiration 81
intra-abdominal sepsis 176–177
intra-aortic balloon counterpulsation
    24–25
  cardiogenic shock 52
intracranial hypertension, critical 11
intracranial pressure (ICP)
  monitoring
    near drowning 230
    traumatic brain injury (TBI) 117
    ventilated patient 111
  normal 112
  raised see raised intracranial pressure
intravenous anesthetic agents 10
  properties 10(fig)
intubation
  diabetic ketoacidosis 144
  pregnancy 262
  smoke inhalation 226
inverse-ratio ventilation 64
iodine 148
iodine-131 (^{131}I) therapy, thyrotoxic crisis
    induction 148
ion exchange resins 101
ionized calcium 153
iron poisoning 248(fig)
ischemic pain, acute myocardial infarction
    42
isoflurane 133(fig)
isoniazid 76, 106(fig)
isoproterenol 26(fig)
isosorbide dinitrate 30(fig)

jejunostomy, percutaneous 199
jugular bulb oximetry 111
junctional tachycardia 31
J waves, hypothermia 232(fig)

Kerley A lines 38
Kerley B lines 38
kidney donors 122(fig)
Klebsiella 70, 73, 74(fig), 77(fig), 138(fig),
    175(fig)

labetalol 28(fig), 259
lactate dehydrogenase (LDH) 44
lactic acidosis
  acute liver failure 166
  massive transfusion 190
Lambert–Eaton myasthenic syndrome (LEMS)
    127
lansoprazole 157(fig)
laryngoscopy, smoke inhalation 226
lead poisoning 248(fig)
left ventricular aneurysm 50
left ventricular assist devices 25
left ventricular end-diastolic volume (LVEDV)
    18
left ventricular failure 35, 37
legal issues 6
Legionella 70, 71, 74(fig), 77(fig), 78(fig),
    175(fig)
lepirudin 90
lidocaine 34(fig)
  status epilepticus 133(fig)
life-sustaining measures, withdrawal 5
limb signs, neurologic monitoring 110
line sepsis 172, 176, 198
lithium carbonate 148
lithium poisoning 248(fig)
liver donors 122(fig)
liver failure, acute 163–167
  causes 163–164
  complications 165–167
  definition 163
  electrolyte disturbances 166
  management principles 164
  metabolic disturbances 166
  presentation 164
  transplantation indications 164–165
liver function tests
  acute liver failure 164
  community-acquired pneumonia 71
  poisoning 239
liver transplantation
  acute liver failure 164–165
  esophageal varices, bleeding 162
living wills 6
locked in syndrome 119
lorazepam 9(fig), 133(fig)

low-molecular-weight heparin 90
Lund and Browder chart 220, 223(fig)
lung collapse
  physical signs 53(fig)
  radiological appearance 54(fig)

macroshock injury 217–218
  consequences 219(fig)
  myocardium 217–218
  nervous tissue 218
  skeletal muscle 218
  vascular tissue 218
magnesium 34(fig)
  tetanus 129
magnesium sulfate
  eclampsia 259
  status asthmaticus 84
malignant hypertension 27, 29
  symptoms 27
  treatment 27, 29
malignant hyperthermia 241
mannitol 113
massive transfusion 188–190
  definition 188–189
  red cell survival 190
  tissue oxygenation 190
mechanical ventilation 61–65
  acute respiratory distress syndrome
    68–69
  cerebral oxygenation 111–112
  clinical applications 61
  clinical assessment 62
  complications 62–63
  diabetic ketoacidosis 144
  GI bleeding risk 159
  Guillain-Barré syndrome 125
  indications 61–62
  liberation from 65–66
    difficulties 65–66
    respiratory function measures 65
  modes 63–64
  neurological function monitoring 110–112
  postoperative 61
  pressure-controlled modes 63–64
  pressure support 64
  status asthmaticus 83–84
  volume-controlled modes 63
meningitis, bacterial 137–139, 177
  antibiotic therapy 138(fig), 139(fig)
  clinical features 137
  diagnosis 137
  treatment 138(fig), 139, 139(fig), 177

meperidine 8 (fig)
metabolic acidosis 93(fig)
  acute liver failure 166
  anion gap 94–95
  hypothermia 232(fig)
  massive transfusion 190
  poisoning 239
metabolic alkalosis 93(fig)
metabolic disturbances
  burns 221(fig)
  hypothermia 232(fig)
  near drowning 229(fig)
  spinal cord injury 216(fig)
methadone 8 (fig)
methanol poisoning 244(fig), 248(fig)
methimazole 148
methylprednisolone
  myasthenic crisis 127
  spinal cord injury 215
  status asthmaticus 83
meticillin-resistant Staphylococcus aureus
    (MRSA) 175(fig), 177, 178, 181
metoclopramide 107(fig)
metronidazole 181
microaggregates, massive transfusion 190
microshock injuries 217, 219
  prevention 219
midazolam 9(fig)
  status epilepticus 133(fig)
milrinone 24(fig)
misoprostol 157(fig)
mithramycin 154
mitral regurgitation 49
Mobitz type I block 48
Mobitz type II block 48
monoamine oxidase inhibitors, poisoning
    249(fig)
montelukast 84
morphine 8 (fig)
  acute renal failure 107(fig)
multiple-dose activated charcoal (MDAC)
    243, 243(fig), 244(fig)
multiple organ dysfunction syndrome (MODS)
    171, 172(fig)
muscle relaxants 10–11
myasthenia gravis
  clinical features 126
  complications 127
  diagnosis 126
  differential diagnosis 126
myasthenic crisis 126
  management 126–127

Mycoplasma pneumoniae 71, 74(fig)
myocardial contusions 207(fig)
myocardial infarction, acute *see* acute
    myocardial infarction (AMI)
myocardium, macroshock injury 217–218
myoclonic seizures 132(fig)
myoglobin 44
myxedema coma 145–147
  cardiorespiratory support 147
  clinical features 145–146
  diagnosis 146
  management 146–147

nafcillin 75(fig), 178
naloxone 240
nasal cannulae 60, 61(fig)
nasogastric suction, pancreatitis 168
nasogastric tubes 199
nasojejunal tubes 199
near drowning 228–231
  clinical features 229
  consequences 229(fig)
  investigations 229
  management 229–230
  outcomes 231
  pathophysiology 228, 230(fig)
near-infrared spectroscopy 112
necrotizing fasciitis 177
Neisseria meningitidis 138(fig), 177
neurological function
  hypothermia 232(fig)
  monitoring 109–112
    ventilated patient 110–112
  near drowning 229(fig)
  poisoning 238
neurologic emergencies 109–139
  see also individual emergencies
neurologic failure, definition 253(fig)
neuromuscular blockade 10–11
  indications 10–11
  organ donors 123–124
nicardipine 259
nifedipine 30(fig)
nimodipine 30(fig), 259
nitrates 30(fig)
  heart failure 39, 40
  unstable angina 41
nitrogen
  parenteral nutrition 200
  requirements 197–198
nizatidine 157(fig)
'no let go' phenomenon 218, 219(fig)

noninvasive monitoring
  cardiovascular system 22–23
  respiratory system 58–59
noninvasive ventilation 64
  chronic obstructive pulmonary disease 86
  status asthmaticus 83
non-Q-wave infarction 44
nonsteroidal anti-inflammatory drugs
    (NSAIDs) 107(fig)
norepinephrine 26(fig)
normothermia, traumatic brain injury 119
nosocomial bacteremia 175–176
  management 176(fig)
nosocomial pneumonia *see* hospital-acquired
    pneumonia (HAP)
nutritional requirements 197–198
nutritional support 197–201
  burns 224–225
  intrinsic renal failure 101
  timing 198
  see also individual support methods

obstetric emergencies 255–262
  see also individual emergencies
omeprazole 157, 157(fig)
opioid analgesics 7–9
  acute renal failure 107(fig)
  acute severe pancreatitis 168
  advantages 8
  disadvantages 8–9
  duration of action 8
  properties 8 (fig)
organ donor management 121–124
  cardiovascular 122–123
  exclusion criteria 121–122
  hematology 123
  homeostasis management 122–124
  intraoperative 123–124
  investigations 122(fig)
  renal 123
  respiratory 123
  temperature 122, 123
organ system failure, definition 253(fig)
oseltamivir 75(fig)
oxygen delivery (DO_2) 55
oxygen therapy 59–61
  acute respiratory distress syndrome 69
  burns 220
  carbon monoxide poisoning 227–228,
    228(fig)
  chronic obstructive pulmonary disease 85
  delivery methods 59–61

pneumonia 72
variable performance devices 59–61, 61(fig)
oxyhemoglobin dissociation curve 59, 60(fig)
carbon monoxide poisoning 227

painless (silent) infarction 42
pancreatitis, acute severe 167–170
causes 167
complications 169–170
diagnosis 167
indications 168(fig)
management 168–169
pathophysiology 167–168
respiratory support 169
surgery 169
panhypopituitarism 150–151
causes 150–151
clinical features 151
diagnosis 151
treatment 151
pantoprazole 157–158, 157(fig)
paracetamol poisoning 244(fig), 245(fig)
paradoxical ventilation 214(fig)
paraldehyde 133(fig)
paraquat poisoning 249(fig)
parenteral nutrition 200–201
acute severe pancreatitis 169
administration 200–201
complications 201
energy requirements 197, 200
feeding regimens 200
intestinal mucosal atrophy 201
parietal cells 156
partial burns 222(fig)
passive regurgitation, aspiration syndromes 79
pathological Q-waves 43
penicillin(s) 178–179
acute renal failure 106(fig)
bacterial meningitis 139(fig)
hospital-acquired pneumonia 77(fig)
pneumonia 74(fig), 75(fig)
pentamidine 75(fig)
pentobarbital 133(fig)
percutaneous gastrostomy 199
percutaneous jejunostomy 199
pericardial effusion 38
pericarditis 49
peritoneal dialysis 102
pethidine 107(fig)
petit mal seizure 132(fig)
phenoxybenzamine 28(fig)

phentolamine 28(fig)
phenylephrine 26(fig)
phosphodiesterase inhibitors 24, 24(fig), 52
pH scale 92
physical examination 2
physical injury 203–236
see also specific injuries
physiotherapy
chronic obstructive pulmonary disease 86
pneumonia 72
piezoelectric transducer 18(fig)
pigmentation, adrenocortical insufficiency 150
piperacillin 179
pituitary function tests 151
pituitary insufficiency 150–151
pituitary macroadenoma 151
plasma osmolality, poisoning 239
plasmapheresis 127
plasma proteins, pregnancy 259(fig)
plasma sodium disorders 134–136, 135(fig)
platelet transfusion
disseminated intravascular coagulation 194
massive 189
pleural effusion
physical signs 53(fig)
radiological appearance 54(fig)
pleural fluid analysis 71
Pneumocystis 75(fig)
Pneumocystis jiroveci (carinii) pneumonia 78–79
pneumonia
antibiotics 74–75(fig)
community-acquired see community-acquired pneumonia
definition 69
health-care-associated 73
hospital-acquired see hospital-acquired pneumonia (HAP)
immunocompromised host 78–79
treatment 78, 79
nosocomial see hospital-acquired pneumonia (HAP)
portosystemic shunting 162
positive end-expiratory pressure (PEEP) 64
acute respiratory distress syndrome 69, 69(fig)
pulmonary barotrauma 62
risk-benefit analysis 3
status asthmaticus 84

posterior cord syndrome 209(fig)
potassium
  diabetic ketoacidosis 143, 143(fig)
  hyperosmolar nonketotic coma 145
  poisoning 239
prednisone 79
pre-eclampsia 255, 258–259
  blood pressure 259
  complications 258
  definition 255, 258
  pathophysiology 258
  risks 255
  treatment 258–259
pregnancy
  acid aspiration syndrome 261
  contraindicated drugs 259
  intubation 262
  physiologic changes at term 255, 256(fig), 257(fig)
  resuscitation 262
  status asthmaticus 262
pressure-controlled ventilation 63–64
processed electroencephalogram (EEG) 112
prokinetic drugs 107(fig)
prone ventilation, acute respiratory distress syndrome 69
propofol 10(fig), 133(fig)
propranolol 28(fig), 148
propylthiouracil 148
prosthetic ventricles 25
protein requirements 197–198
  intrinsic renal failure 101
Proteus 73, 77(fig), 177
proton pump inhibitors (PPIs) 156, 157–158, 157(fig)
  interactions 158
Pseudomonas 74(fig), 81
Pseudomonas aeruginosa 73, 139(fig), 175(fig), 176(fig)
pulmonary artery catheters (PACs) 18–22
  cardiac output measurement 20
  cardiogenic shock 51
  complications 20(fig)
  data derived 19(fig)
  hemodynamic variables 21, 22(fig)
  indications 21, 22
  insertion 18
  perioperative use 22
  thermodilution 20
pulmonary artery flotation catheter (PAFC) 20, 168

pulmonary artery wedge pressure (PAWP) 18, 20
  sources of error 21(fig)
pulmonary barotrauma 62
pulmonary damage, smoke inhalation 226–227
pulmonary edema 88
pulmonary embolectomy, acute 92
pulmonary embolism (PE) 87–92
  clinical features 88
  decision-making guidelines 89
  etiology 87
  hemodynamic profile 27(fig)
  investigations 88–89
  pathophysiology 88
  size 88
  thrombolytic therapy 91–92
  treatment 90–92, 90(fig)
pulmonary hyperinflation, status asthmaticus 83–84, 84(fig)
pulmonary tuberculosis see tuberculosis, pulmonary
pulmonary venous hypertension 38
pulse oximetry 58
  carbon monoxide poisoning 227
pupils
  asymmetry 109–110
  brain death 121(fig)
  neurological function monitoring 109, 111(fig)
  poisoning 238
pyrazinamide 77
pyridostigmine 127

Q-wave, pathological 43

rabeprazole 157(fig)
raised intracranial pressure 112–115
  acute liver failure complication 165
  causes 113
  clinical features 113
  encephalopathy 165
  management 113
Ramsay sedation scale 11, 11(fig)
ranitidine 157(fig), 168
recombinant tissue-type plasminogen activator (rtPA) 90(fig)
regional analgesia, sedation reduction 13
renal failure
  acute see acute renal failure (ARF)
  acute liver failure complication 166
  definition 253(fig)

renal impairment
  burns 221(fig), 224
  hypothermia 232(fig)
renal resuscitation protocol 99–100, 100(fig)
renal support
  acute 102–107
  acute severe pancreatitis 169
respiratory acidosis 93(fig)
  poisoning 239
respiratory alkalosis 93(fig)
  poisoning 239
  pregnancy 262
respiratory failure
  acute-on-chronic 85
  aspiration syndromes 81
  causes 67–69
  definition 253(fig)
  management 67
  perioperative 57
  pregnancy 262
  smoke inhalation 226–227
  traumatic brain injury 118
  type I (acute hypoxemic respiratory failure)
      56, 67
  type II (ventilatory failure) 56–57
  type III (perioperative) 57
  type IV (shock with respiratory muscle
hypoperfusion) 57
respiratory muscles
  atrophy, mechanical ventilation 62
  innervation 213(fig)
respiratory system 53–95
  acute liver failure 166
  burns 221(fig)
  hypothermia 232(fig)
  near drowning 229(fig)
  noninvasive monitoring 58–59
  poisoning 238
  pregnancy 258(fig)
resuscitation
  cardiac arrest 35, 36(fig)
  esophageal varices, bleeding 160–162
  poisoning 240–241
  pregnancy 262
rewarming, hypothermia 233–234
  active core 234
  active external 234
Richmond Agitation Sedation Scale 11, 12(fig)
rifampicin 74(fig)
rifampin 77, 181
right ventricular end-diastolic volume (RVEDV)
      17, 19(fig)

right ventricular failure 37
rimantadine 75(fig)
risk-benefit analysis 3
rule of nines 220

salbutamol 26(fig)
Salmonella typhi 176(fig)
sclerotherapy, endoscopic 161
scoring systems 251–254
secondary heart block 48
second degree burns 222(fig)
sedation 7–13
  complications 12
  daily interruption 12–13
  indications 7
  reassessment 2
  reduction 12–13
  requirements 11
seizures
  control, traumatic brain injury 119
  etiology 130–131
sepsis 171–172, 172(fig)
  acute renal failure 102
  causes 176–178
  intra-abdominal 176–177
septic shock 27(fig)
shock
  burns 219, 232
  cardiogenic see cardiogenic shock
  hemodynamics 27(fig)
  septic 27(fig)
  spinal 213, 214, 215
  traumatic 205
sickle cell β-thalassemia 186(fig)
sickle cell disease 186–188, 186(fig)
  acute crises 187
    management 188
  features 186–187
  sequestration 187
sickle cell disorders 185–188, 186(fig)
  incidence 185
  laboratory diagnosis 186
  pathophysiology 185–186
sickle cell hemoglobin C disease 186(fig)
sickle cell hemoglobin D disease 186(fig)
sickle cell trait 185–186, 186(fig)
silent (painless) infarction 42
simple partial seizure 132(fig)
single-dose charcoal 241
sinus arrest 49
sinus brachycardia 49
skeletal assessment, poisoning 238

skeletal muscle, macroshock injury 218
skin assessment, poisoning 238
smoke inhalation 225–228
  clinical features 225
  management 226–228
  prognosis 228
sodium
  diabetic ketoacidosis 143
  disorders 134–136, 135(fig)
sodium bicarbonate 101
sodium nitroprusside 30(fig)
  cardiogenic shock 52
  pre-eclampsia 259
  pregnancy 259
solid material aspiration 80
somatostatin 161
spastic paralysis 215
spinal cord injury (SCI) 208–216
  above C3 lesions 214(fig)
  above C5 lesions 212, 214(fig)
  assessment 208–209
  C5-C8 lesions 214(fig)
  chronic post-transection period 215, 216(fig)
  clinical evaluation 208
  C6 lesions 212
  early hospital management 209–215
    airway 209–211, 212(fig)
    breathing 211–213
    circulation 213–214
    spontaneously breathing patient
      212–213
  field management, immediate 209
  gastrointestinal system 216(fig)
  immobilization 209, 215, 215(fig)
  neurosurgical management 215
  primary 208
  radiology 209, 210(fig)
  secondary
    pharmacological treatment 215
    prevention 208
  syndromes 209(fig)
  T1-T6 lesions 214(fig)
  T7-T12 lesions 214(fig)
  ventilatory support indications 212
spinal reflexes, brain death 119
spinal shock 213, 214, 215
splanchnic ischemia 155
splenic injury 206
spontaneous breathing trials 66
sputum sampling
  community-acquired pneumonia 71
  hospital-acquired pneumonia 174

Staphylococcus aureus 73, 75(fig), 77(fig),
  78(fig), 81, 176(fig)
starvation, hypercatabolic response vs. 198(fig)
status asthmaticus
  features 83
  immediate management 83
  intensive care 83
  mechanical ventilation 83–84
  pregnancy 262
status epilepticus 130–134
  causes 131
  classification 132(fig)
  complications 134
  investigations 134
  management 132–133, 133(fig)
  pseudostatus 131
  stages 132(fig)
  supportive treatment 132
steroid hormones 149
steroids
  acute respiratory distress syndrome 69
  chronic obstructive pulmonary disease 86
  dosage guide 152(fig)
  hypercalcemia 154
Stewart–Hamilton equation 20
Streptococcus 73, 176(fig)
Streptococcus agalactiae 138(fig)
Streptococcus pneumoniae 70, 75(fig),
  138(fig), 175(fig), 187
Streptococcus viridans 177
streptokinase 46, 90(fig)
stress ulcer formation 155
subclavian vein catheters 16(fig)
succinylcholine 107(fig)
sucralfate 157(fig), 158
sudden death 47–48
sulfamethoxazole 75(fig), 79, 181
sulfonamides 106(fig)
superficial burns 222(fig)
suprasternal cardiovascular monitoring 22
supraventricular arrhythmias 29, 31
supraventricular tachyarrhythmias, organ
  donors 123
supraventricular tachycardia (SVT) 29, 31
synchronized DC cardioversion 29
synchronized intermittent mandatory
  ventilation (SIMV) 63
syndrome of inappropriate antidiuretic
  hormone secretion (SIADH) 134, 136
  causes 136
  clinical features 135(fig)
  treatment 135(fig)

systemic embolism 49, 207(fig)
systemic inflammatory response syndrome
    (SIRS) 171–172, 171(fig), 172(fig)
  burns 224

temperature
  organ donor management 122, 123
  poisoning 238
  transfused blood 189
tension pneumothorax 207(fig)
tetanospasmin 128
tetanus 128–129
  clinical features 128, 128(fig)
  complications 129
  diagnosis 128
  differential diagnosis 128
  management 128–129
  neuromuscular blockade 11
  prognosis 129
therapeutic goals, defining 3
thermal injury
  electrical 217
  smoke inhalation 225
thiopental 113
third degree burns 222(fig)
thoracic electrical bioimpedance 23
thrombi
  acute myocardial infarction 41
  formation 87, 87(fig)
thrombin 192
thrombocytopenia 194
thrombolytic therapy
  acute myocardial infarction 45
    drug choice 47–48
    indications 45
  acute renal failure 107(fig)
  complications 46, 91
  contraindications 45–46, 91(fig)
    absolute 45, 91(fig)
    relative 45–46, 91(fig)
  pulmonary embolism 91–92
thrombotic crisis, sickle cell disease 187
thymoma 126
thyroid disorders 145–149
thyroid function tests 146(fig)
thyroid replacement therapy
  dose 146
  myxedema coma 146–147
  regimens 147
thyroid stimulating hormone (TSH) 145
thyrotoxic crisis 147–149
  causes 147–148
  clinical features 148
  management 148–149
  metabolic management 148–149
thyroxine (T_4) 145
  thyroid replacement therapy 147
tissue donors 122(fig)
tissue oxygen tension (PO$_2$), sickle cell
    disorders 185–186
tocolytic-induced pulmonary edema 260
tonic-clonic epilepsy 132(fig)
torsade de pointes 35
total calorie intake 197
toxicology 237–249
  ABC 240
  active treatment 241
  antidotes 244, 244(fig), 245–249(fig)
  clinical assessment 237–238
  co-ingestions 237
  drug elimination increasing measures
    241–244
  history 237
  ICU admission criteria 241
  investigations
    non-toxicological 239–240
    toxicologic 240
    trial by antagonist 240
  management 240–244
  resuscitation 240–241
tracheal intubation, spinal cord injury 209–211
tracheostomy 66
  emergency
    smoke inhalation 226
    spinal cord injury 211
transcranial Doppler, ventilated patient 112
transesophageal echocardiography 23
transfusion
  burns 224(fig)
  massive see massive transfusion
  sickle cell disease 188
transfusion reactions 188–192
  acute hemolytic 190–191
  definition 188
  non-hemolytic 191–192
    grading 192(fig)
transjugular intrahepatic portosystemic
shunt (TIPS) 162
transplant coordinator 121
transthoracic echocardiography 23
trauma
  airway management 203, 204(fig)
  breathing 204
  breathing assessment 204

circulation 205
  fluid management 207
  management principles 203–206
    emergency assessment 203
    primary survey 203
    secondary survey 203
traumatic brain injury (TBI) 115–119
  artificial ventilation 118
  conduct of transfer 116–117
  deep vein thrombosis 119
  initial management 115
  intracranial pressure monitoring 117
  intubation/ventilation indications 116
  neurosurgical center transfer indications 116
  positioning 118
  repeat scan indications 118
  secondary management 117–118
traumatic shock 205
treatment, reassessment 2–3
tricyclics, poisoning 249(fig)
triiodothyronine (T₃) 145
  thyroid replacement therapy 147
trimethoprim 181
  acute renal failure 106(fig)
  pneumonia 75(fig), 79
troponin I 44
troponin T 44
Trousseau's sign 152
tuberculosis, pulmonary 76–78
  clinical features 76
  diagnosis 76
  management 76–78
  risk factors 76
T-wave inversion 43

unstable angina see angina, unstable
upper airway
  obstruction, smoke inhalation 225
  thermal injury 221(fig)
urea
  acute renal failure 99
  community-acquired pneumonia 71
  poisoning 240
urinalysis
  acute renal failure 99
  poisoning 239
urinary tract infections 177
U-tube manometer, fluid-filled 18(fig)

valganciclovir 182
vancomycin 181
  acute renal failure 106(fig)

bacterial meningitis 138(fig), 139(fig)
  pneumonia 75(fig)
variable performance devices, oxygen therapy
  59–61, 61(fig)
vasoactive drugs 3, 161
vasoconstrictors 24
vasodilation, heat stroke 234
vasodilators 30 (fig)
vasopressin 161
vasopressors 24
Vaughan-Williams classification,
  antiarrhythmic drugs 31(fig)
vecuronium 11
venous puncture, central venous
  catheterization 17(fig)
ventilation, inadequate 205(fig)
ventilation, mechanical see mechanical
  ventilation
ventilator-associated pneumonia (VAP)
  clinical features 173
  definition 173
  diagnosis 76(fig), 78, 173–174
  treatment 174, 175(fig)
ventilatory failure 56–57
ventricles, prosthetic 25
ventricular afterload reduction 40
ventricular arrhythmias 35
ventricular fibrillation 35
  acute myocardial infarction 48
  microshock injuries 219
ventricular obstruction 37
ventricular preload reduction 40
ventricular septal defect, acquired 49–50
ventricular tachycardia (VT) 35, 49
ventricular volume overload 37
Venturi mask 61(fig)
verapamil 30(fig), 31, 34(fig)
viral hepatitis 163
viral infections, pneumonia 75(fig)
Virchow's triad 87, 87(fig)
vitamin D deficiency 151
vitamin K, warfarin reversal 91
volume-assured pressure support 64
volume challenge 2
voriconazole 183

warfarin
  acute myocardial infarction 47
  pulmonary embolism 90
  reversal 91
warming, organ donor 122, 123
wound management, burns 224

X-rays
  abdominal, poisoning 240
  chest *see* chest X-ray

Zollinger–Ellison syndrome 162–163